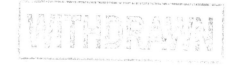

D0363883

OXFORD MEDICAL PUBLICATIONS

Friendly Fire
Explaining Autoimmune Disease

Even the finest weapons are instruments of great evil.
Lao Tzu

Friendly Fire
Explaining Autoimmune Disease

David Isenberg

Professor of Rheumatology
Bloomsbury Rheumatology Unit/
Division of Rheumatology
Department of Medicine
University College London

and

John Morrow

Senior Lecturer in Immunopathology
Department of Immunology
The Medical College of Saint
Bartholomew's Hospital
University of London

OXFORD   NEW YORK   TOKYO
OXFORD UNIVERSITY PRESS
1995

Oxford University Press, Walton Street, Oxford OX2 6DP
Oxford   New York
Athens   Auckland   Bangkok   Bombay
Calcutta   Cape Town   Dar es Salaam   Delhi
Florence   Hong Kong   Istanbul   Karachi
Kuala Lumpur   Madras   Madrid   Melbourne
Mexico City   Nairobi   Paris   Singapore
Taipei   Tokyo   Toronto
and associated companies in
Berlin   Ibadan

Oxford is a trade mark of Oxford University Press

Published in the United States
by Oxford University Press Inc., New York

© David A. Isenberg and W. John W. Morrow, 1995

A catalogue record for this book is available from the British Library

Library of Congress Cataloging in Publication Data
Isenberg, David.
Friendly fire : explaining autoimmune disease / David A. Isenberg
and W. John W. Morrow.
p. cm.—(Oxford medical publications)
Includes index.
1. Autoimmune diseases—Popular works.   I. Morrow, W. John, W. 1949–
II. Title.   III. Series.
[DNLM: 1. Autoimmune Diseases—popular works. WD 305 178f 1995]
RC600.I84   1995   616.97'8—dc20   94–46700
ISBN 0 19 262220 X

Typeset by Footnote Graphics, Warminster, Wilts.
Printed in Great Britain by
Bookcraft (Bath) Ltd, Midsomer Norton

Preface

When we are children our bodies seem both natural and, most of the time, in perfect working order. It is only gradually that we come to appreciate the remarkable harmony and integration of the various organs and systems that enable us to grow up and grow old.

In many societies there is an expectation of good health. Serious illness is often hard to accept, or is ascribed to forces outside our control. The truth is both more remarkable and rather different. However, understanding the nature of disease requires us to understand how the body works and protects itself normally. Although such knowledge has increased enormously in the past 50 years, nevertheless we remain relatively ignorant of how the single cell from which we start our lives is converted into the organism made up of many billions of interacting cells. How do these cells learn their lines and play their roles? Why, in some people, do these cells fail to fulfil these roles—with unpleasant and even tragic consequences? The mechanisms involved are still being worked out, but the roles at least are much better defined. Clearly a very important function is that of self-defence.

Over the countless years of evolution very sophisticated processes have developed to defend the body; these processes have a dual purpose. There are 'enemies' both without and potentially within the body. Thus the immune system has evolved to ensure that foreign microbes can be recognized and speedily destroyed. But the system also has a watching brief over the body's own tissues to ensure that, for example, cancers will not develop and destroy the organism. The immune system thus consists of a veritable army of cells, especially in the blood and lymphatic systems, whose functions are to perform these two roles.

Increased public awareness and curiosity about diseases of the immune system (considerably heightened by the catastrophic impact of AIDS) has prompted us to write this book. Unfortunately, while illnesses such as rheumatoid arthritis, diabetes, and multiple sclerosis occur all too often, how they originate seems obscure and poorly understood.

We have attempted to analyse how the body defends itself and what the consequences are when that defence system—the immune system—loses control and attacks itself. Military metaphors have been hard to resist but will not, we hope, be too distracting. Friendly fire is the phrase used to describe the unfortunate events that may follow when a military force inadvertently attacks its own combatants, mistaking them for the enemy. By analogy, autoimmune diseases result when an immune system mistakenly attacks the body's own healthy tissues. Our main goal is to explain the nature of self-destructive or autoimmune diseases and so to demystify the immune system and convey our own sense of fascination for the process of biological discovery. Being forced to write without the crutch of scientific jargon has been a humbling experience! This has been a necessary and probably long overdue change. We wish to thank Lucy Isenberg, Ann Maitland, Liz Carr, Marilyn Over, and especially Eleanor Flood for their assistance. We also thank Ann Maitland for typing much of the manuscript, Professor Tony Pinching for constructive criticism, and the staff of the Oxford University Press, who encouraged us in the belief that this was a book worth writing.

This is a book for the general reader who may lack a formal scientific background but who wants to know how the human body defends itself—and to understand the illnesses which result when it fails to do so.

February 1995   D. A. I.
                                                                 W. J. W. M.

Contents

1

What exactly is the immune system—and what does it have to do with disease?

The immune system: a description of what it is, how it works, and what happens when it malfunctions form the basis of this book. It is perhaps a sign of the times, a legacy of the AIDS epidemic, that public awareness of the immune system is greater than ever before. Almost daily it seems that the news media have something to say about antibodies, killer cells, or CD4/CD8 ratios. The jargon is endless! In fact, the immune system is a highly complex defence network that defends us from bacteria, viruses, and other infectious micro-organisms, which can enter the body and cause disease, and protects against the development of other disorders, such as cancer. It comprises a veritable army of cells whose function is to protect the body by remaining vigilant and eliminating such 'intruders' when necessary. To perform this crucial function the immune system has at its disposal an arsenal which easily rivals that of any army in sophistication and scope. Recruitment procedures, communication networks, repair mechanisms, as well as long and short range 'weapons of destruction' are all part of the body's militia.

The function of the immune system

Probably without realizing its scientific significance, most of us will have been aware of our immune system from an early age. We are vaccinated for protection against common viruses and bacteria, a practice that usually begins at around 6 months of age, and which can leave strong impressions! Again without understanding the process, we acquire immunity when we catch diseases such as mumps and measles. Where no effective vaccine is available, the spread of childhood diseases such as chicken pox is often encouraged '. . . to get them over and done with'. Thus we learn that the immune system has its own 'memory', and that once it has come into contact with, and responded to, an organism foreign to the body it can remember the invader and deal with subsequent attacks very rapidly, in many cases resulting in the complete elimination of the organism. A state of active immunity is thus maintained for life. This state of permanent protection is based on the ability of the immune system to differentiate between 'foreign' material (non-self) and the body's own tissue (self). The ability to make this distinction is crucial.

Immunodeficiency

In the main the immune system does an admirable job. However, like any piece of machinery, it can go wrong. Immunodeficiency occurs when an individual's immune system does not function normally and recognize micro-organisms that have entered the body. This failure may cause disease if the 'invaders' are not destroyed. Immunodeficiency may occur because of faults due to inherited (genetic), microbiological, or environmental factors. It can have dire consequences, notably overwhelming infections. Some individuals are born with a condition that leads to immunodeficiency, others acquire diseases, such as AIDS, that, for different reasons, have the same immunodeficient effects.

Autoimmune (self-destructive) diseases

Immunodeficiency diseases are not the only form of immunological failure. There are circumstances when the immune system fails to recognize the body's own components as 'friendly' and mounts an attack on these 'self' tissues.

In this book we will use the term autoimmunity in two senses:

- To describe a state in which the immune system of an individual allows the production of antibodies (types of protein) or the activation of cells which react with components of the body's own tissues. This state, as will become clear, is not a rare phenomenon, but is carefully controlled in a healthy individual.
- To describe the consequence of these defects which combine with other factors to cause the development of abnormal symptoms and physical signs. Thus autoimmune diseases are the direct result of damage to the body's own tissues by the defence mechanisms which, under normal circumstances, protect the body but which have now 'turned traitor'. Unfortunately, disorders of this type are relatively common and include rheumatoid arthritis, juvenile (insulin-dependent) diabetes, thyroiditis, and multiple sclerosis.

What causes autoimmune diseases?

Many diseases are caused by self-destructive processes—it seems that none of the body's organs or systems is safe from potential attack. What remains puzzling is why some individuals suffer from autoimmune diseases while others, often close relatives (including on occasion an identical twin) can escape. Autoimmune diseases are the result of a combination of different factors going wrong at the same time. These factors include:

- an inherited (genetic) predisposition;
- hormonal influences;
- abnormalities in enzymes found in the blood;
- stress;
- diet;
- ultraviolet light;
- micro-organisms (notably bacteria and viruses).

It seems very likely that the same sorts of factors are involved in causing autoimmune diseases as seemingly different as multiple sclerosis and rheumatoid arthritis. By rearranging these factors in different ways, various diseases may develop (see Chapter 4).

A short history

Our understanding of autoimmunity is closely linked to what we now know about the functioning of the normal immune system. While it took thousands of years before man could do anything other than simply contemplate the way in which the body protects itself from infection, the last 30 years have seen spectacular advances in our knowledge of the structure and function of the immune system.

For many centuries it was assumed that all human diseases were simply variations upon some common theme. It was not until the sixteenth century that European physicians began to accept that there are large numbers of different diseases. It is therefore only in the past 500 years that diseases such as bubonic plague, smallpox, syphilis, and malaria have been recognized as distinct entities, and only in the past 35 years that the full extent of the self-destructive autoimmune diseases has been recognized.

Thomas Sydenham, a seventeenth-century English doctor, appears to have been the first to recognize that diseases were classifiable, but it was not until the eighteenth century that attempts were made to categorize diseases, and it was over 100 years before this aim was successful. It was also during the eighteenth century that the first notions of preventive medicine were put to a form of clinical trial by Edward Jenner, a family physician in the village of Berkeley, Gloucestershire. There had been some previous attempts (in Turkey and ancient China, for example) to inoculate against smallpox. However, it was Jenner who noticed that dairymaids who suffered a minor condition called cowpox seemed never to develop smallpox. By deliberately inoculating individuals with cowpox, Jenner was able to show that they could indeed develop immunity to the much more serious, life-threatening smallpox. The government of the day was so impressed by these results that Jenner was awarded grants of £10 000 and £20 000 to develop his work. Allowing for 200 years' worth of inflation, the present value of these awards must be over £1 million! However, it has been suggested, perhaps cynically, that the government, although worried about the effects of recurrent epidemics of smallpox on the population as a whole, was more concerned about ensuring sufficient numbers of healthy young men to maintain its army at full strength!

Considering how many other infectious diseases are now treated by immunization, it was a nice quirk of fate that (in 1977) smallpox itself became the first infectious disease to be eradicated world-wide.

By the beginning of the twentieth century, the idea of completely separate diseases with different causes and treatments was widely accepted, and medical research began to focus on just how the body protects itself under normal circumstances. Studies of infectious disease have led to the identification of cells that normally protect us against viruses and bacteria. Gradually, and only relatively recently, has it come to be realized that the same cells could malfunction and cause havoc.

In common with many other facets of medicine, the recognition of autoimmunity has been hampered by 'statements of the famous'. Such pronouncements are too often based on insufficient information and prejudice but acquire an aura of authority and come to represent formidable barriers to understanding. There are numerous examples of this type of obstacle in science and medicine, ranging from the problems experienced by William Harvey in the seventeenth century in persuading the medical profession to accept the circulation of blood from the heart around the body, to the wild assertions of the geneticist Trofim Lysenko. This Russian scientist made outlandish claims to have converted late ripening into early ripening wheat and also to have transformed wheat into rye. Tragically, his political patronage by Stalin resulted in the disgrace and death of scientists who doubted his claims and set back Soviet agricultural genetics for two decades.

In the field of autoimmunity, a major barrier to progress was inadvertently erected by one of the luminaries of immunological research, Paul Ehrlich, who doubted that the immune system would permit the development of 'anti-self' components:

> The organism possesses contrivances by means of which the immunity reaction, so easily produced by all kinds of cells, is prevented from acting against the organism's own elements and so giving rise to autotoxins. Further investigations made by us have confirmed this view, so that one might be justified to speak of a 'horror autotoxicus' of the organism. These contrivances are naturally of the highest importance for the existence of the individual.

The idea that the immune system would react against host, or 'self' tissue was therefore dismissed by researchers in the early 1900s. They considered the body incapable of reacting with 'internal elements' (i.e. with itself) but also noted that 'when internal regulating contrivances are no longer intact, great dangers can arise'. This astute and basically correct observation (that the body is regulated internally and that disorders in this regulation can cause serious problems) triggered many attempts to explain the great mystery of the immune system—namely, its ability to generate specific responses to an apparently infinite number of foreign substances, and also its ability to discriminate between 'self' and 'non-self'. Although many theories were proposed, they were all unconvincing, and a plausible explanation for these aspects of immunoregulation was lacking for half a century.

It is paradoxical that, at the time he wrote of the unlikelihood of the body permitting a reaction against itself, Ehrlich himself provided one of the first descriptions of a clinical autoimmune disease—an uncommon condition known as paroxysmal cold haemoglobinuria. Ehrlich noted that, by placing a tourniquet around the finger of a patient with the disease and immersing the finger first in cold and then in warm water, he caused destruction of red blood cells and leakage of haemoglobin (the pigment that gives red blood cells their colour) into the urine (with its subsequent discoloration).

Other early descriptions of what turned out to be autoimmune diseases were made by Widal and colleagues, and Chauffard and Troisier, who, during the first decade of the twentieth century, identified several forms of haemolytic anaemia (destruction of red blood cells). However, by this time, the notion of Ehrlich's 'horror autotoxicus' (i.e. the impossibility of 'anti-self' components) was so strongly held that the evidence produced by these and other authors was largely ignored. Indeed it was not until

1945, when Robin Coombs, working in Cambridge, developed a reliable technique to detect the presence of antibodies to red blood cells, that the concept of autoantibodies (antibodies that bind to 'self' tissue) gained recognition. Within a few years, antibodies to red blood cells were recognized as being responsible for the damage caused by haemolytic anaemia.

In the early 1950s, researchers in the UK (Ivan Roitt and Deborah Doniach), the USA (Noel Rose and Ernest Witebsky), and New Zealand (Duncan Adams) were able to prove the existence of autoimmune thyroid disease. The studies published by these researchers, in 1956, were to prove a landmark in the recognition of self-destructive disease. Within a year of the recognition of this first organ-specific autoimmune disease came the simultaneous description by four laboratories of antibodies binding to DNA in patients with systemic lupus erythematosus, a generalized auto-immune condition. In 1960 John Simpson, a Scottish neurologist, suggested that myasthenia gravis (a condition causing variable muscular weakness, now known to be the result of damage at the junction of muscle and nerve fibres) might also be an autoimmune condition. The list of probable autoimmune diseases has expanded rapidly as shown below:

- Diseases mainly affecting one organ/system (organ specific):
    diabetes mellitus;
    Hashimoto's thyroiditis (underactive thyroid);
    Graves' disease (overactive thyroid);
    pernicious anaemia;
    primary biliary cirrhosis;
    chronic active hepatitis;
    autoimmune haemolytic anaemia;
    autoimmune thrombocytopenia (low platelet levels);
    pemphigus;
    multiple sclerosis;
    myasthenia gravis;
    myositis.
- Diseases affecting several organs/systems (non-organ specific)
    systemic lupus erythematosus;
    rheumatoid arthritis;
    Sjögren's syndrome;
    scleroderma.

Thus, within a short period of time the very concept of 'horror autotoxicus' was challenged and has subsequently been turned on its head, as it has become clear that, far from being abnormal, the production of antibodies that bind to self-components or self-antigens is probably the rule. For example, in many individuals with simple infections of the bladder or the bloodstream (septicaemia) a wide range of autoantibodies can (temporarily) be found. Cells grown from blood in the umbilical cord of newborn children have the capacity to produce autoantibodies. It is also possible to produce from normal adults an array of monoclonal (highly purified) antibodies which bind to different self components. However, these 'autoimmune phenomena' are usually well controlled by the body and do not cause harm. It is only when they get out of hand and the factors referred to earlier in the chapter interact that an autoimmune disease develops.

Prevalence and frequency of autoimmune diseases

Accurate estimates of the number of people with autoimmune disorders are difficult to obtain. The number of individuals in a given population with a particular disease at any one time is referred to as the disease prevalence. This is often calculated by assessing the number of cases in a known area such as a city, and multiplying the number on a per capita basis so that it applies to the whole country. However, this can be in-accurate as it does not take account of environmental influences and variations in ethnic groups, which may be spread unevenly around the country. For example, thalassaemia, a disease affecting the red blood cells, is very common in the Cypriot population and hence common in parts of north London but rare in other parts of the UK.

Other problems bedevil attempts to obtain really accurate figures of just how common a condition actually is. For example, criteria used to diagnose a disease have changed over time, especially as new laboratory tests have become available. Opinions of the importance of certain clinical features have also been revised in some cases. For example, Raynaud's phenom-enon (a condition in which the hands and feet go through distinct white, blue, and red colour changes in response to cold or occasionally emotion) used to be considered an important diagnostic feature of systemic lupus erythematosus. However, it has become obvious that while many patients with systemic lupus erythematosus have Raynaud's phenomenon, a majority of the individuals who experience this temperature sensitivity do not have lupus. In addition, Raynaud's phenomenon is now known to occur in a variety of other conditions. It has therefore been removed from the list of criteria needed to make a diagnosis of lupus.

Differences in prevalence of disease amongst ethnic groups are well illustrated by systemic lupus erythematosus which occurs in approximately 1:250 black women (in the USA), 1:1000 Chinese women, and 1:4300 white women (figures from New Zealand). In other cases where ethnic differences at first sight appear to be important, closer examination of the facts suggests that other influences are being brought to bear. Thus rheumatoid arthritis which has a prevalence approaching 1:100 in white people is very rare amongst the rural black population in South Africa. This might be interpreted as being due to a racial difference. However, studies have shown that when this rural population moves to the local towns (for example to Soweto, near Johannesburg) the prevalence of rheumatoid arthritis increases dramatically to become virtually the same as that of the adjacent white population. In this case the evidence favours an environmental factor such as an infectious agent being responsible for triggering the disease in a relatively overpopulated town.

It is of great interest that certain Native North American tribes, such as the Yakima and the Chippewa, are between three and five times more likely to develop rheumatoid arthritis than the local Caucasian (white) population. This could be interpreted as an ethnic difference but may also be due to an infectious agent more common amongst these tribes.

There is considerable variation in the development of individual auto-immune diseases at different ages. As an example, insulin-dependent diabetes invariably begins before the age of 20. There are also some notable fluctuations in prevalence of certain diseases according to geographical location. Thus those living in northern Scotland are approximately 40 times more likely to develop multiple sclerosis than those living on the south coast of England. This sort of variation has yet to be fully explained.

In most European countries and the USA, it is realistic to say that at least 5 per cent of the population (i.e. 1 in 20) will suffer from a self-destructive autoimmune disease during their lifetime.

The cost of autoimmune disease

There are no precise figures concerning the cost of looking after patients with autoimmune diseases. However, the Middlesex Hospital, London has estimated that an average medical outpatient clinic visit (based on 1994 figures) costs around £50. A course of treatment inflates this figure to at least £100 per attendance. Assuming that patients with rheumatoid arthritis and diabetes are reasonably representative of the medical outpatient population, it is possible to make some informed estimates of how much it costs to look after patients with autoimmune diseases.

Most patients whose rheumatoid arthritis or diabetes is stable will be assessed four times per year. They will invariably be on regular treatment. Thus for both of these common disorders, it must cost at least £400 per year in terms of outpatient hospital visits. As these patients will need to continue treatment from their family doctors in between hospital visits, costs will effectively be doubled – at least £800 per year. Assuming a combined prevalence of rheumatoid arthritis and diabetes of 1 per cent of the UK population (which is approximately 55 million), about 550 000 individuals must suffer from these two diseases. Even if we assume that only half of these patients are attending hospital and/or receiving adequate treatment, the health bill for outpatient care can be estimated at £220 million per year. Although some patients with rheumatoid arthritis and diabetes are seen less frequently than four times per year, the reduced costs of looking after these patients will be balanced by those with active disease, who are seen more frequently and who require multiple drugs. In Britain the total cost of looking after patients with diabetes has recently been estimated at about 5 per cent of the NHS budget (£1.2 billion per year). Most of this sum is spent on managing complications of the disease. A few years ago in the United States, the cost of looking after patients with diabetes was estimated at $10 billion.

The figures quoted above exclude all the other autoimmune diseases, some of which, like systemic lupus erythematosus, are by no means rare and require much more frequent hospital outpatient assessment. On balance, therefore, it is reasonable to suggest that the total outpatient bill for autoimmune diseases in the UK is very likely to exceed £1000 million. As the population of the USA is approximately four times that of the UK, and as USA medical costs appear to be higher, it seems likely that their outpatient bill will be in the region of £5000 million (about $7500 million).

However, this is only part of the story, as many patients with auto-immune diseases require costly inpatient hospital treatment. The Bloomsbury Rheumatology Unit, London, has estimated (1994 figures) that the total cost of having a patient in a hospital bed for an average 2- to 12-day stay is just over £1000. It is difficult to generalize about the numbers of patients with autoimmune disorders who are hospitalized. From our own experience, about 5 per cent of patients with rheumatoid arthritis are hospitalized once per year. Excluding the costs of operations (a frequent reason for admission), and assuming that there are 300 000 patients with rheumatoid arthritis in the UK, there may be around 15 000 rheumatoid arthritis hospital admissions (or 'episodes') per year. In 1994 these cost say, £1000 each, gave a total cost of approximately £15 000 000 for that year. This calculation excludes the costs of severe arthritis sufferers who require long-stay hospital treatment. These figures serve to emphasize that autoimmune diseases have profound economic as well as personal consequences. The cost of caring for the victims of these self-destructive diseases is truly phenomenal!

2

How does the immune system actually work? The components

The immune system comprises a veritable army of cells which can be activated to fight off challenges from all manner of foreign invaders. In this chapter we will review the structure and function of the immune system. Specifically we will:

- Examine the organs concerned with the body's defence.
- Review the cell types found in the immune system organs as well as in the blood and discuss their function.
- Contemplate how the components of the immune system work together to eliminate foreign invaders.

How does the immune system work?

In Chapter 1 we described briefly the immune system and mentioned that it had many similarities to an army, as Peter Parham has pointed out. Now we will consider this analogy in further detail. As with any military organization, new recruits have to be trained to perform certain specialized functions, and are then posted to various locations where they can best carry out their duties. As well as sharing some of the same goals and aspects of organization and day-to-day operation of a real-life defence force, the immune system shares its strengths and weaknesses. Thus, they are both:

- able to function against selected targets;
- large, complicated, and elaborate;
- subdivided into distinct compartments which perform apparently identical functions;
- prepared for events that may never happen;
- liable to fight today's threats with solutions of past problems;
- able to destroy that which they protect;
- susceptible to corruption;
- slow to react;
- costly;
- wasteful.

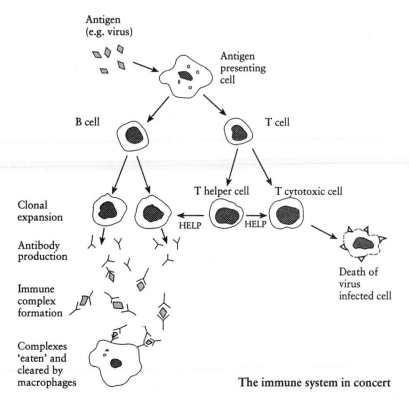

Figure 2.1. When the body is attacked, the immune system responds by challenging and defeating the invader. The invader (antigen) is arrested by a presenting cell such as a macrophage and is partially digested before being handed over to the B cells and T cells for identification. T helper cells, produced by the T cells, produce cytokines, which enhance the B cells' antibody response by signalling that they produce more antibody. (If the invader, in this case usually a virus, is presented directly to the T cells, cytotoxic (killer) T cells will be generated.) Once triggered, the B cells transform into antibody-producing plasma cells and manufacture the specific antibody, which binds to the antigen and triggers the complement system. The complement system recruits neutrophils to help eliminate the antigen, perhaps with additional help from macrophages.

Both armies and the immune system can be readily mobilized to fight off external threats or to maintain internal order. Mostly they perform this task well and are very successful at 'repelling invaders' but a high price has to be paid for maintaining this constant vigilance. The immune system, like an army, is expensive (biologically) to support and most of the time enjoys a relatively tranquil existence, not engaged in combat.

Furthermore it can be heavy-handed and error-prone in its operation, and in some cases resorts to mutiny. Such a mutiny is the principal topic of this book.

Following an intrusion or attack to the body by a foreign 'invader' or antigen (for example bacteria, viruses, or toxins) the components of the immune system co-operate to challenge and defeat the threat. Briefly, cells 'on patrol' in the blood 'apprehend' the invaders, identify them, and then mobilize certain specialized cells (different antigens require distinct treatment) whose function it is to neutralize and destroy the attackers (see Figure 2.1).

The organs of the immune system

The immune system operates throughout the entire body. However, certain organs are involved more closely with the immune system than others.

The lymph system

The foot soldiers of the immune system are the different types of white blood cells produced in the bone marrow and the lymph glands.

Bone marrow

The bone marrow can be likened to a recruitment centre—it collects young, untrained individuals and organizes them for general and then specialized training in one of several military disciplines. Blood cells originate in the bone marrow. All blood cells have a common ancestor—known as a stem cell—a primitive type of cell that may be likened to a new teenage recruit. Like its human counterpart, the stem cell is unsure of its role within the environment, can be moulded relatively easily by external influences, and is driven by a very powerful desire to reproduce! Stem cells, while having no specific function, divide rapidly and are converted into several types of white blood cells.

Lymph glands

Lymph glands occur throughout the body. They are linked by a system of vessels (lymphatic vessels), which carry a specialized fluid—lymph. This fluid contains only one type of cell—specialized white blood cells known as lymphocytes.

Other organs involved in the production of white blood cells

Thymus

The thymus, which is located near the junction of the chest and neck, is primarily a training camp for lymphocytes. It is here that lymphocytes (which were produced in the bone marrow and travelled via the lymph system to the thymus) are trained in their crucial roles in the organization of the body's defences. Training results in two types of thymus-derived lymphocytes (T cells):

- helper T cells;
- suppressor/cytotoxic T cells.

Which type of T cell a lymphocyte becomes depends on the influence of various hormones present in the thymus at the time of training.

Tonsils and spleen

Not all the lymphocytes produced in the bone marrow travel to the thymus. Other important training camps are the tonsils, spleen, and various patches of lymphoid tissue in the gut. In these areas, lymphocytes are turned into B lymphocyte cells (B cells) and become responsible for making antibodies. (B cells derive their name from the Bursa of Fabricius, an organ found in the rear portion of the gut in birds.)

The cells of the immune system

The blood contains two major types of cell, which can be categorized on the basis of their colour:

- red blood cells;
- white blood cells.

Red blood cells

Red blood cells (also known as erythrocytes) are vitally important. They carry oxygen from the lungs to the other parts of the body and perform several other vital functions. However, they are of limited interest to immunologists because they are not involved in defence functions.

White blood cells
The second category of cell found in the blood is the white cell population. These comprise a relatively small percentage of the overall bulk of cells in the blood but, nevertheless, it is these cells that delight and confound immunologists. While these cells were first identified in the blood, hence the name, it is important to remember that many of them, especially the lymphoid cells, are also present in the body tissues. Indeed it is in the tissues that white 'blood' cells can cause much mischief. The white cells can be subdivided into three groups—lymphocytes, macrophages, and neutrophils.

Lymphocytes

T cells
The thymus-derived T cells comprise three-quarters of the circulating lymphocytes. These cells have many important functions regulating immune reactions, of which the principal ones are:

- facilitating or enhancing immune responses;
- suppressing immune responses.

Enhancement of immune responses
Once an attacking foreign invader (the antigen) has been arrested, it is handed over to the T cells and B cells, which are responsible for producing and co-ordinating the precise response to this particular invader. T helper cells enhance the production of antibodies—the bullets of the immune system—by the B cells. Antibodies attack and destroy the invading antigen. The antibody response is always specific to the particular antigen.

Suppression
Other T cells function as cytotoxic (killer) or suppressor cells. This kind of response is particularly useful in dealing with virus infections and cancer cells. The T suppressor cell can 'damp down' certain immune responses at an appropriate time. For example, if the immune system responds to an offensive microbe, such as the gut bacterium *Salmonella*, and eliminates it from the body within a few days, then there is no longer a need for the continued production of *Salmonella* antibodies. Suppressor cells will act to shut down the production of *Salmonella* antibodies. They may do this by releasing soluble factors—messenger molecules—which act on the B cells to reduce their output of antibodies. Alternatively, they may knock out cells involved in immune reactions more directly.

The different types of T cells can be identified by the presence of certain molecular structures on their surfaces. The helper cell population bears a 'flag' or marker called CD4 (CD stands for 'cluster of differentiation'); the cytotoxic suppressor cell group can be recognized by the presence of a molecule called CD8. The CD4 and CD8 molecules can be used as convenient synonyms for the T helper and T cytotoxic/suppressor cells.

B cells

The B cells are the front line infantry of the immune system. They make up approximately one-quarter of the circulating lymphocytes and their function is to produce antibodies, the primary ammunition of the immune system (see below). The way in which the immune system has evolved to manufacture antibodies that react only with a certain specific microbe or toxin is intriguing. This is the concept of antigen-specificity and is a recurring theme in immunology. The ability of antibodies to react with a vast number of different foreign organisms depends largely upon their capacity to recognize different three-dimensional structures associated with each of these organisms. There are two possibilities as to how the immune system produces an antibody to a specific antigen; the problem can be illustrated by considering a man wanting to buy a suit:

- He can go to a tailor, who will measure his size, cut the cloth, and make the suit to fit him.
- He can go to a big store with thousands of ready-made suits and simply try them on until he finds the best fit.

In the same way, the immune system could have developed a tailor-made approach, i.e. wait until the foreign organism 'comes in', 'size it up', and then manufacture a specific antibody to destroy it. In reality the immune system has evolved to use the 'big store' approach. Thus it has available literally hundreds of millions of antibodies, from which the 'best fit' is selected.

The B cells that produce the required antibody are encouraged to multiply by a mechanism called clonal expansion (see Figure 2.2). In this process, the specific B cells capable of producing the appropriate antibody are activated but, prior to making the antibody, they divide. The increased population of specific B cells is then transformed into plasma cells, which are geared towards producing large amounts of antibody. These responses ensure that enough antibody is produced to deal with the offending antigen. The plasma cells have a relatively short life (only a few weeks). After they have fulfilled their antibody-producing function, they die. The death

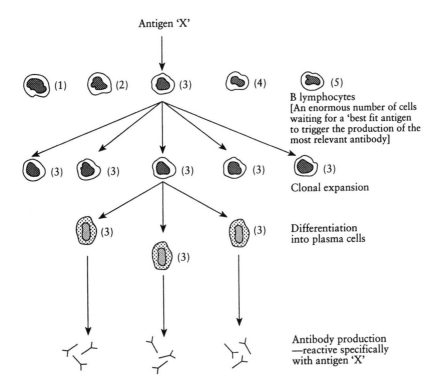

Figure 2.2 Clonal expansion of the B cell population in response to an antigenic stimulus. The numbers 1 to 5 represent different types of B lymphocytes.

of the plasma cells shrinks the expanded B cell population back to its original size. In other words, the population expands to combat the presence of infection and contracts once this task is accomplished.

Macrophages
Macrophages are very important multipurpose cells in the immune arsenal. They are distributed throughout the body, in the tissues as well as the blood (those found in the blood are more correctly called monocytes). A most important function of macrophages is the ability to 'present' antigen to other components of the immune system.

Antigen presentation
It is the macrophages that seize on intruding antigens (invaders) and present them, after first digesting them with enzymes that break down proteins, to B cells and T cells, thus initiating a series of essential immune

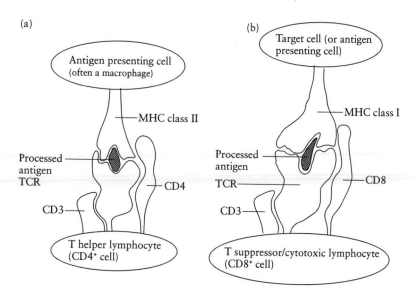

Figure 2.3 Schematic representation of antigen processing.

responses. The scheme of antigen presentation, which is fundamental to all specific responses, is outlined in Figure 2.3.

An important facet of this process is that the antigen is presented to the T cells together with a complex of structures on the cell surface. This is called the major histocompatibility complex (MHC), and it determines the type of response to the antigen. Depending on the nature of the initial immune response from the T cells and B cells, the antigen can be accompanied by class I or class II major histocompatibility complex molecules. The major histocompatibility complex molecules are placed in these categories for several reasons although these are somewhat complicated; essentially the classification is due to their biological and physical characteristics although further description is outside the scope of this book. There is also a third class of major histocompatibility complex molecules, but these are esoteric species, even for immunologists, and we will make no further mention of them here.

Typically, antigens that are presented with class II major histocompatibility complex will be delivered to T helper cells (T cells with the CD4 marker) and an antibody response results. Antigens that associate with class I molecules are normally presented to cytotoxic/suppressor T cells (with the CD8 marker) and a cytotoxic response results. It is important to note that the responding population of T cells recognizes the combined shape of the antigen and the major histocompatibility complex molecule. The combination of T cell receptor, major histocompatibility complex molecule, and antigen fragment is known as the trimolecular complex. As there is some variation in the appearance of the major histocompatibility complex molecules due to genetic variation, some antigens may be more effective than others in inducing immune responses because they present an optimum shape or conformation to the T cells.

In man, the major histocompatibility complex molecules are also called human leucocyte antigens or HLA. Human leucocyte antigen molecules are distributed throughout the body tissues and it is through differences in this system that cells are classified as self or non-self. The human leucocyte antigen class I molecules can be subdivided into three main categories (HLA-A, HLA-B, and HLA-C) while the class II molecules have several categories (e.g. DR, DP, DQ). The human leucocyte antigen molecules vary considerably from person to person. For example, there are approximately 50 known variants of HLA-B. Each individual has a combination of molecules from all these human leucocyte antigen categories on the surface of the cells in their body and, given the great variation between individuals, the possibility of two individuals having the same combination of human leucocyte antigen molecules is very remote. It is this particular aspect of the immune system that presents problems for organ transplantation. Unless the human leucocyte antigen type of the donor and the recipient are virtually identical, the organ graft will not 'take'—that is it will be rejected by the immune system of the host. The process of tissue typing involves the identification of the set of human leucocyte antigen antigens in the tissues of a given individual.

Phagocytosis

Other macrophages have a phagocytic role—they consume passing antigens —and thus act rather like immunological vacuum cleaners. Macrophages, unlike T cells or B cells, do not bind to any particular structure (i.e. they lack specificity); and therefore do not react with the same precision as T cells or B cells. However, macrophages are equipped with various features that make them particularly effective at removing foreign antigens. On their surface they have receptors that recognize specific structures on the tail end of antibody molecules and so can intercept, catch, and dispose of complexes of antigen bound up with antibody. In this regard they have been called 'professional phagocytes', a term that distinguishes them from other cells that can ingest micro-organisms in special circumstances. Such cells, which include endothelial (which form the lining of blood and lymphatic vessels) and epithelial (or surface) cells as well as fibroblasts (found in the connective tissue), are sometimes called 'non-professional' phagocytes.

Granulocytes

Granulocytes are another type of white blood cell, so-called because of the granules they contain. Several types of granulocytes are involved in the immune response. They are all produced in the bone marrow and are relatively short lived. The most important of these are the neutrophils which are also known as polymorphonuclear cells — the latter name reflecting the fact that the nucleus of these cells has a rather shapeless form with distinctive multiple lobes.

Neutrophils

Neutrophils may be thought of as the SAS commandos or the Delta Force of the immune system and high levels of these cells in the blood point strongly to the presence of infection. However, they tend to be heavy-handed and frequently cause damage to innocent tissues in their haste to deal with the threat to the body; they are certainly not 'smart weapons'.

Neutrophils circulate in the blood and eliminate invaders by phagocytosis. Like macrophages, they are non-specific in their *modus operandi*. They travel quickly to the site of any tissue injury or immune reaction (recruited by various chemical signals) and can participate in many immunological reactions. Large numbers of neutrophils cause the inflammation seen at the site of an injury. In particular, neutrophils are known for releasing an enzyme that is particularly toxic to micro-organisms. Neutrophils can be found anywhere in the body where there is a need for a very rapid, active, immune response.

Eosinophils

Another cell of the granulocyte family is the eosinophil. These cells appear to be used selectively for parasitic infections. Unlike neutrophils, they do not appear to be phagocytic but they contain many large granules, easily visible under a microscope, which are an important part of their weapons system. On contact with the parasite target the eosinophil releases its granules rather like a cluster of hand grenades. Eosinophils appear to be particularly effective in combating nematode (worm) parasites.

Basophils, mast cells, and platelets

Basophils are involved in inflammation although this role is rather obscure. Mast cells appear rather similar under the microscope: their best recognized function is an involvement in allergic reactions. Another cell in this family is the platelet or thrombocyte. Platelets have several functions, mostly involved with blood clotting and wound healing. Although they do not perform antigen-specific immunological functions, they are important in inflammatory processes. In addition, there are several diseases in which the platelet is subjected to autoimmune attack.

Substances made by the immune system

The cells of the immune system manufacture and release into the blood a large number of substances that regulate responses. Broadly speaking these materials can be categorized into three groups as follows.

Antibodies

Antibodies are perhaps the most well-known and best studied elements of the immune system. They are the bullets of the defence forces (or perhaps mini cruise missiles, as they home-in on their targets) and are manufactured and used in enormous quantities.

Antibodies are made by plasma cells. For the purposes of biological economy, the structure of each antibody molecule is essentially similar, except for the areas that determine its specificity. Thus, the factors that determine whether an antibody will bind to an influenza virus or to a *Salmonella* toxin can be found as distinctive structural features in relatively small regions of the antibody. When assembled, the complete antibody molecule is Y-shaped. A schematic representation of an antibody is shown in Figure 2.4. Antibodies, also called immunoglobulins, can be classified according to certain structural characteristics or their particular functions. Once an antibody has bound to a given antigen, an immune complex is formed. Immune complexes have many biological properties. Mostly they are formed as part of the process of antigen elimination however they can also have effects that are deleterious to the body. We will consider these negative characteristics further in Chapters 3 and 4.

Cytokines

Once activated by an antigen, macrophages secrete messenger molecules called cytokines to give additional warning and stimulate the immune

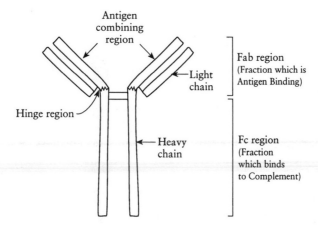

Figure 2.4 Schematic diagram of an antibody molecule.

system to deal with an impending antigen threat. Essentially, cytokines are manufactured by lymphocytes or other immune cells and released into the bloodstream. Once they reach their destination (usually a cell) they induce a specific biological effect. This effect varies according to the cytokine and the cell involved but, typically, cytokines signal certain cell populations to activate themselves, divide, or home-in on a particular site in the body.

Interferon

One of the first cytokines discovered was interferon. In the early 1960s, a sensational future was predicted for this molecule and, indeed, one of the first clinical trials was described in a Flash Gordon cartoon (see Figure 2.5)! Unfortunately, as is often the case in medical research, the antiviral effects of interferon that were evident in test tube experiments proved to be somewhat more complicated in living animals. Nevertheless, the interferon genes have now been isolated (cloned) by modern molecular biology techniques and large quantities can be produced by cells 'engineered' and grown for this purpose. In fact there is a family of interferon molecules, called alpha, beta, and gamma. Some of these products, particularly interferon-alpha, are being used to treat life-threatening diseases of humans, including cancer.

Certain technological breakthroughs have made cytokine research a 'hot topic' for immunologists over the last decade. Specifically, these advances have come through the very powerful techniques of molecular biology. Scientists working in this field have discovered how to identify and isolate genes responsible for the production of specific protein molecules.

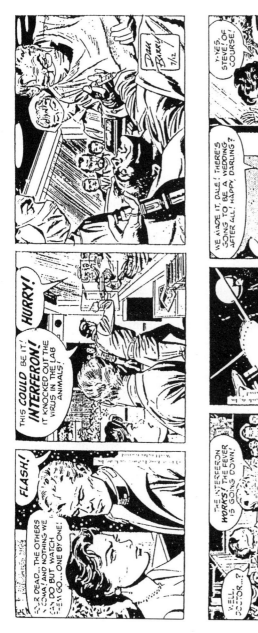
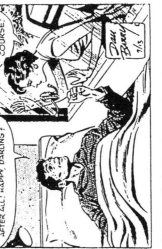
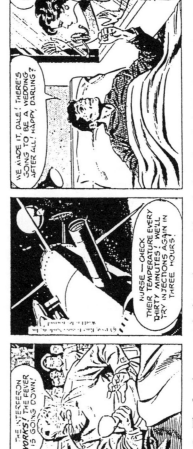

Figure 2.5 The first human trial of interferon as 'described' in the Flash Gordon comic strip (copyright 1960: King Features Syndicate).

Molecular biology has almost limitless prospects that have ramifications for all aspects of biomedical research. Naturally genetic engineering (the process by which genes are manipulated to obtain a desired biological product) has been applied to immunology and more specifically, cytokine research, and many factors have been isolated, cloned, and characterized; some have been found to have clinical as well as research applications. Examples of such clinical applications are the recent production of large quantities of monoclonal antibodies to different targets e.g. those binding CD4 molecules and the cytokine known as TNF alpha which are now being used to treat patients with rheumatoid arthritis and Crohn's disease (see Chapter 6).

Complement

The complement system is a series of enzymes that act in a sequential order with antibodies to remove bacteria and other organisms to which the antibody molecule is attached. Essentially, there are nine major components of the system, although some of these fragment into smaller pieces, which can act in their own right. Unfortunately, the nomenclature of the complement system is confusing—the numbers designated to the various components were given in their order of discovery. Some time after naming, it was found that the components of the complement system did not interact in this order!

The complement system, which works through two main pathways, has several important functions in the normal immune system. In particular it helps to activate macrophage cells, to destroy unwanted cells, and to prepare (opsonise) bacteria for digestion by phagocytic cells (Figure 2.6).

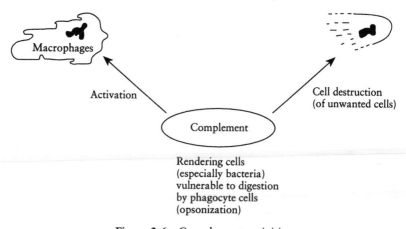

Macrophages

Activation

Cell destruction
(of unwanted cells)

Complement

Rendering cells
(especially bacteria)
vulnerable to digestion
by phagocyte cells
(opsonization)

Figure 2.6 Complement activities.

The complement system is relevant to autoimmune diseases for two major reasons. First, complement becomes involved in autoimmune reactions and can have a very damaging effect on host tissues. Second, deficiencies of complement (usually for genetic reasons) may predispose individuals to the development of systemic lupus erythematosus and certain types of infectious diseases.

3

What has to go wrong before an autoimmune disease develops? The factors involved in autoimmunity

Autoimmune disease can result from several different defects, or combinations of defects, in the immune system. In this chapter we will review:

- Defects that occur in the immune system and predispose an individual to an autoimmune condition.
- Defects that arise following infections.
- Genetic predispositions to autoimmunity.
- The influence of hormones, diet, drugs, and ageing on the development of autoimmunity.

Defects in the immune system

There is little doubt that autoimmune disease arises as the result of a complex interplay of factors. It is now an established fact that individuals are born with a greater or lesser predisposition to developing an auto-immune disease. It is also clear that women are at greater risk of develop-ing virtually every kind of autoimmune disease. Differences in the risk of acquiring these disorders have also been shown to vary according to ethnic background, although environmental factors, such as exposure to different bacteria or viruses, must also be taken into consideration when examining any racial basis of disease. The exposure to different infections, diet, stress, ultraviolet light, and chemical toxins are all contributing factors to auto-immune disease.

Like any other part of the body, defects can arise in the immune system. These disorders fall into two broad categories:

- Immunodeficiency—when the immune system does not recognize invaders as being undesirable and therefore does not mobilize to destroy them.
- Autoimmunity (self-destruction)—when the immune system fails to recognize 'self' as friendly and mounts an attack on itself.

Very early in life, most of the cells that could react with the body's own tissues are eliminated or, in the immunologist's terminology, clonally deleted. However, this process does not guarantee that the immune system will not, in various circumstances, turn nasty and attack the body that is its host. In fact autoimmunity can be caused by abnormalities or defects in almost any part of the immune process.

Abnormalities of B cells

Abnormalities of the B cells play a key role in the defence of the body by producing antibodies. The immune system reacts to threats from viruses, bacteria, and other 'foreign' micro-organisms in a highly specific manner. Following a challenge from an invading micro-organism (antigen), the B cells produce antibodies that bind to the intruder. The complex of antibody and antigen (in this case a part of the intruder) is then removed. One of the simplest ways of proving the importance of a particular cell or its product(s) is to look at those unfortunate people who, for one reason or another, lack the ability to produce them. In this respect B cells are particularly important because a wide variety of different clinical syndromes is associated with their absence or impaired functioning. As indicated, the inability of B cells to produce normal quantities of antibodies is associated, as might be predicted, with an increased risk of infection. In addition, patients have an increased risk of developing an autoimmune disease.

The importance of B cells and the antibodies that they produce, as well as being illustrated by a complete or relative absence, is also emphasized when a single antibody-secreting B cell (plasma cell) becomes malignant and produces an excess of unwanted antibody. The excess antibody can often bind to parts of the 'self' (self-antigens), including DNA, thyroid tissue, and white blood cells. Indeed, in a recent study in our laboratory, approximately one-third of such antibodies were found to be capable of binding to one form of self-antigen or another. This proportion was much higher than had previously been thought likely, and indicates that self-tissues and foreign invaders may often have partially similar structures. However, the production of antibodies that bind to self-antigens is only one factor that predisposes to autoimmune disease and, alone, is insufficient to cause the clinical features of an autoimmune disease. Thus none of the patients we have studied has had any evidence of such a disorder.

Autoantibodies

Most self-destructive diseases are associated with the presence, often in substantial quantities, of antibodies that are capable of binding to 'self' components (autoantibodies). As discussed on page 5, Paul Ehrlich originally put forward the view that the body would not permit the development of such autoantibodies under normal circumstances, and thus their presence would only be associated with autoimmune diseases. In the past 20 years, however, it has become established that a wide variety of autoantibodies can be detected in the serum of perfectly healthy individuals. It is now certain that the mere production of antibodies that can bind to a 'self' component will not alone cause the clinical features of an autoimmune disease.

Autoantibodies in healthy individuals

Studies of B cells have suggested some important distinctions between the autoantibodies found in the blood of patients with autoimmune disorders and those found in the blood of healthy people. Perhaps one of the most important of these differences is that the autoantibodies found in healthy people tend to bind rather weakly to their target antigens, and indeed may react with a wide variety of seemingly different structures. This apparent 'polyreactivity' may be explained by the sharing of a small surface component by otherwise different antibody molecules. By analogy, compare a flower pot to a top hat: these very different items have similar shapes and may be the same size (see Figures 3.1 and 3.2).

Autoantibodies in autoimmune disease

Antibodies binding 'self' components as part of an autoimmune disease tend to bind much more tightly to their respective antigens. Good examples of such autoantibodies are those that bind to DNA, which are found in patients with systemic lupus erythematosus, and those that bind to the acetylcholine receptor that are found only in patients with severe myasthenia gravis.

Types of B cell

The surfaces of most cells within the body are covered with molecular structures, or markers (as described on page 16). These markers enable us to identify different groups of cells. This concept is also true of the B cells and, within the past few years, a particular set of B cells has been identified because they all carry the so-called CD5 marker, which has been shown to have a particular relevance to autoimmune diseases. These cells form a large proportion of the total number of B cells before birth. Increased numbers of these CD5 B cells are also present in patients with rheumatoid arthritis, juvenile chronic arthritis, and Sjögren's syndrome. Approximately 25 per cent of patients with rheumatoid arthritis have this

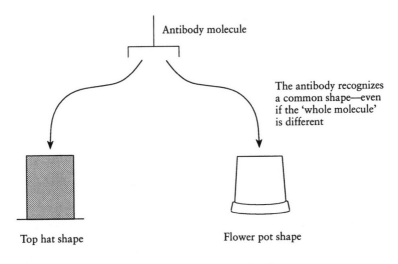

Antibody molecule

The antibody recognizes a common shape—even if the 'whole molecule' is different

Top hat shape

Flower pot shape

Figure 3.1   Antibodies recognize shapes.

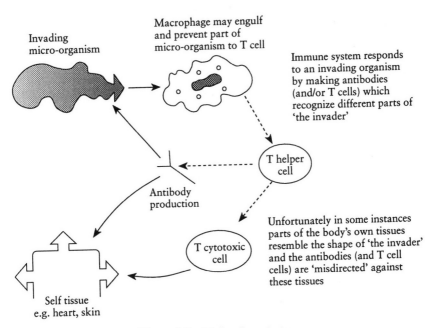

Invading micro-organism

Macrophage may engulf and prevent part of micro-organism to T cell

Immune system responds to an invading organism by making antibodies (and/or T cells) which recognize different parts of 'the invader'

T helper cell

Antibody production

T cytotoxic cell

Unfortunately in some instances parts of the body's own tissues resemble the shape of 'the invader' and the antibodies (and T cell cells) are 'misdirected' against these tissues

Self tissue e.g. heart, skin

Figure 3.2   Molecular mimicry.

marker, compared with 10 per cent or fewer of healthy individuals. Studies from a number of laboratories have indicated that CD5 B cells have a predisposition to produce antibodies that bind to single-stranded DNA and produce rheumatoid factors.

Abnormalities of T cells

The immune system contains several types of white blood cell one example of which is the lymphocyte. One of the populations of lymphocytes, the T cells, can be further divided into:

- T suppressor cells;
- T helper cells.

T suppressor cells

The function of the T suppressor cells is to regulate the body's response to antigens and thus to keep the immune system in check. T suppressor cells are also thought to be responsible for distinguishing between 'self' and foreign tissues, and thus they prevent autoimmunity. There is evidence to suggest that patients with autoimmune diseases have poorly functioning T suppressor cells. This implies that these individuals are more likely to develop a self-destructive (autoimmune) disease because their immune system has a reduced ability to regulate itself when challenged by foreign, or even 'self', components.

Research studies

The 1970s and early 1980s saw a lot of research (using animal models of human diseases) into the actions of these T suppressor cells. For example, the New Zealand black/white mouse (which suffers a disease closely resembling human systemic lupus erythematosus) was found to have a reduction in the number and function of T suppressor cells. Furthermore, the development of kidney disease in these mice has been found to correspond to a further deterioration in T suppressor cell function. It can be assumed that a similar sequence of events takes place in individuals whose T suppressor cells show qualitative or quantitative deficiencies.

Experimental autoimmune encephalitis, which is an animal model for multiple sclerosis, can be produced in laboratory rats. In this model too, a defect in T suppressor cell function is present. This defect has been shown to be inherited, as inoculation of other types of rat does not produce the disease. T suppressor cell defects have also been reported in other animal models of autoimmune diseases, such as spontaneous auto-immune thyroiditis in chickens.

Autoantibody production

It is widely believed that the seemingly unregulated autoantibody production in human autoimmune disease is the result of inadequate T suppressor cell function. Thus decreased numbers and activity of T suppressor cells in patients with virtually all types of autoimmune disorders have been reported. Intriguingly, abnormalities in T suppressor cell function have also been identified in some otherwise healthy relatives of systemic lupus erythematosus patients. This finding is further confirmation that there are important genetic components of autoimmune conditions and that, as with B cells, T cell malfunction alone is insufficient to cause an auto-immune disease.

Thus, T suppressor cell function is the result of a balance of different influences. Any disturbances in this delicate balance may well upset the regulation of B cells by T cells (via the cytokines produced by the helper T cells), which in turn influences the production of autoantibodies that can act against the individual's own immune system.

T helper cells

Just as a deficiency of correctly functioning T suppressor cells may pre-dispose an individual to autoimmune disease, so might an excess of T helper cells. Under normal circumstances these cells enable the immune system to make an effective response to any given antigen. This is done by certain structures on the surface of T helper cells called the class II molecules. The function of these molecules is to present antigen to the appropriate cells (in this case B cells) so that an antibody response can be generated. It is now known that an excess of class II molecules is present in individuals with autoimmune syndromes. This situation could, theoretic-ally, lead to an excess of T cell help, i.e. an over-production of self-antigens. The expression of class II molecules is under genetic control and increased levels of these molecules, while not causing disease as such, increase the susceptibility of the individual to autoimmunity.

Complement deficiency

Another factor that may lead to the development of an autoimmune dis-ease is a deficiency of certain components of the complement system. The complement system is a complicated system of enzymes whose primary task is to assist in the removal of antigens that have been trapped by antibodies. It is therefore activated after an antibody has combined (com-plexed) with an antigen. The generation of such antigen–antibody com-plexes is a normal part of the immune response and the complexes are cleared from the circulation by macrophages; if not cleared efficiently, inflammation and autoimmunity can result.

One of the main functions of complement is to dissolve (or 'solubilize') antibody–antigen complexes. However, deficiencies in certain components of the complement system may prevent this solubilization. Complete or even partial absence of the second component (C2) of complement is a major risk factor for developing autoimmune disease, in particular systemic lupus erythematosus and myositis. Inherited deficiencies of the other complement components are less common but many have been described and all are associated with an increased tendency to develop autoimmunity.

Infection

Given that the immune system is constantly being challenged by infectious agents, it is not surprising that occasionally some of these organisms can take advantage of a defect in the system and, on occasions, 'trigger' autoimmune conditions. There are many examples of infectious organisms causing temporary abnormalities of the immune system and signs and symptoms typical of autoimmune diseases.

Inflammation

The influenza virus will cause fever, swollen lymph glands, and aching muscles. Infection with the rubella virus (German measles) is sometimes the cause of swollen and painful joints. Many of these symptoms arise from the inflammatory events, such as antibody–antigen complex formation, which occur as the immune system attempts to eliminate the virus. However, the symptoms are short-lived and the diseases are self-limiting. Thus self-destructive events can arise from infections if the immune system does not eliminate the invading organism quickly and efficiently and if other predisposing factors are present.

AIDS

A good example of how the immune system fails to cope with an invader is acquired immune deficiency syndrome (AIDS). It is now clear that the human immunodeficiency virus (HIV)—the virus that causes AIDS—can induce many long-lasting symptoms including arthritis, thyroiditis, diabetes, thrombocytopenia, Sjögren's syndrome, and other disorders that resemble 'classic' autoimmune disease. Furthermore, the events leading to the catastrophic collapse of the immune system that characterizes AIDS are probably due to a self-destructive 'civil war', which occurs as the body's defence system makes frantic and mostly ineffective attempts to neutralize the infection.

Over-reaction of the immune system to infection

Another illustration of how the immune system can inflict grave damage on the body is its occasional heavy-handed treatment of infections such as measles, which can result in inflammation of the brain (encephalopathy).

A further example is the damage done as the immune system attempts to overcome a small parasite—*Trypanosoma cruzi*—that infects the nervous system. The immune system sends many cells towards the site of these infections and, in their attempts to destroy the invading parasite, these cells also cause considerable damage to the surrounding, non-infected 'innocent' tissue. In the case of *Trypanosoma cruzi* infection, the damage to the nerves in the arms and legs leads to weakness and muscle wasting. A real-life analogy is the damage caused by fire fighters as they extinguish a fire—it is quite common for the water damage to exceed the destruction caused by the fire itself! In addition considerable damage may be caused by the fire fighters in their attempts to gain access to the fire.

Molecular mimicry

Molecular mimicry is an important concept in the relation between infection and autoimmunity. It refers to a situation when part of the structure of an invading microbe resembles some component of the host's body tissues. In other words, certain infectious organisms can trick the immune system into attacking parts of the host's body because of a superficial resemblance. A good example of this is rheumatic fever. Following an infection with streptococcal bacteria, susceptible patients develop abnormalities in one of their heart valves because their immune system cannot distinguish the microbe and certain tissues associated with the valve.

Heat shock proteins

In relation to molecular mimicry, there has recently been a great deal of interest in heat shock proteins—a family of proteins found originally in cells that had been subjected to high temperatures (although they have since been found to appear in response to a variety of stressful stimuli, including starvation and infections). It is now known that heat shock proteins exist in all cells at normal temperatures and have several important functions. These include helping to transport other proteins around the cell and preserving the cell's protein structure during times of stress.

Because many heat shock proteins have been conserved through evolution they are very similar in shape to organisms as diverse as bacteria and man. It has been suggested that the immune response to heat shock proteins in micro-organisms could result in autoimmunity if the immune system mistakes these proteins on the surface of the invading bacteria for the body's own heat shock proteins. The potential for such a reaction occurring would be greatly enhanced if heat shock proteins were present in abnormally high numbers.

Autoimmunity and infection

Further links between autoimmunity and infection have been provided by studies of patients with viral, bacterial, and parasitic infections. Many patients infected with common micro-organisms, as well as producing antibodies against the micro-organism, also make autoantibodies that bind to DNA, to the cell wall of red blood cells, and other self tissues. Conversely, patients with autoimmune disease have frequently been reported to have high levels of antibodies that recognize various microbes.

However, the interpretation of these observations is subject to what might be called the 'Clouseau' principle. This relates to an episode in the 'life' of the famous fictional French detective. On chasing a suspect into a small hotel he observed a large dog standing between the hotel proprietor and the door through which the suspect had fled. 'Monsieur,' inquired the Inspector, 'Does your dog bite?' 'Non! my dog does not bite,' replied the proprietor. Clouseau then attempted to get past the dog ... and was promptly bitten. 'I thought you said your dog does not bite,' shouted the angry Inspector. 'Monsieur,' the proprietor informed him, 'this is not my dog!' In other words, two observations—the presence of the disease and the detection of certain antibodies in patients with the disease—do not prove that one is the cause of the other. The association might be circumstantial rather than causative. For example, patients with an autoimmune disease may, at the same time, be exposed to an infecting agent. The immune system may also be more susceptible to a given microbe—due to a defect within the system. Alternatively, an antibody that is produced by the immune system because it recognizes some part of an infecting antigen might, by chance, also be able to bind to a self-antigen.

Cancer

There are a number of links between autoimmune diseases and cancer. In certain situations cancer and autoimmunity may occur simultaneously. For example, both dermatomyositis, especially in males over the age of 50, and Sjögren's syndrome are thought to be associated with an increased risk of developing certain tumours, although, certainly in the case of dermatomyositis, this risk is relatively small. In addition, rheumatoid arthritis has been linked to an increased chance of developing cancer of the lymphatic tissues with a relative risk (i.e. the chance of an individual being studied developing a given disease compared with the general population) of between 2.7 and 15 times.

Studies that have attempted to link autoimmune disease and malignancy have been beset with difficulties. For example, it has been argued that the association of two diseases (autoimmunity and malignancy) may be subject to statistical distortion if the diagnosis of one condition makes the diagnosis of another more likely. In other words, the association between the two may be a form of self-fulfilling prophecy because patients with an autoimmune disease will be screened much more extensively than a patient without such a disease, thus increasing the chance of discovering a malignancy. There is also a major problem in terms of identifying suitable populations for comparison and a further difficulty in that many of the immunosuppressive drugs that are used to treat patients with autoimmune diseases may themselves be responsible for the development of cancer.

Oncogenes

Studies of cancer and self-destructive disorders suggest that common mechanisms may underlie both types of disease. Indeed, one link between autoimmunity and cancer has been demonstrated by the discovery of oncogenes (genes that are capable of converting normal cells into cancerous cells). It has been claimed that the roots of cancer lie in our genes. Cancer has been shown to begin with changes in the DNA of a particular gene in a particular cell. The cell then multiplies relentlessly and its descendants form a large mass of cells called a tumour. The tumour often grows and so prevents normal body functions.

One school of thought has suggested that 'silent' (inactive) oncogenes might be present in all cells—perhaps acting under normal circumstances to help control cell replication—and that activation of these silent genes by viruses, carcinogens, or environmental factors might then produce a malignancy.

In an update of this theory it has been confirmed that oncogenes are altered versions of normal genes, which in normal cells act as central regulators of growth. During life a variety of changes could convert one of these normal genes into an oncogene. However, the development of a single oncogene, while perhaps necessary for the development of a tumour, is by itself insufficient. The development of cancer, like autoimmune disease, requires multiple steps.

Much work has been done to suggest that viruses, particularly retroviruses, can infiltrate the body's cells and 'switch on' an oncogene. Recent evidence has shown that patients with active systemic lupus erythematosus have increased production of certain oncogenic proteins.

In some respects autoimmune diseases may be thought of as the consequence of a malignant process. Thus lupus is characterized by the long term proliferation of certain B cells, while rheumatoid arthritis is associated with a massive overgrowth of synovial cells that line certain joints. It is tempting to speculate that part of the 'immunological fire' that burns in patients for so many years may be fuelled by oncogenes.

Other genetic influences

To date, oncogenes have been detected in about 20 per cent of human tumours. This may be partly because methods for detecting them are, as yet, unsophisticated. However, this observation has prompted many studies for other genetic factors that may in part be responsible for the development of malignancies.

One major area of research concerns the existence of certain genes whose function seems to be to suppress growth. These genes are important because they restrict the growth of cells. Clearly, then, mutant forms of such growth suppressor genes might allow the unrestricted growth of cells. Furthermore because, at least in theory, mutant forms could be found in sperm or ova (eggs) they might be passed from one generation to the next. This in turn might explain the observation that certain types of cancer 'seem to run in families'. Such a mechanism might also be relevant to the development of autoimmune diseases in several members of the same family.

The links between autoimmunity and cancer are further emphasized by another group of tumours known as the lymphomas. Lymphomas are malignancies derived from the B cells before they have been 'converted' into antibody secretors. They are thus derived from stem cells and represent 'solid' tumours of the immune system. Patients with lymphomas are often unable to respond to certain foreign antigens. These patients may thus be more susceptible to infection.

Lymphoma is a recognized late complication of some patients with rheumatoid arthritis, Sjögren's syndrome, and systemic lupus erythematosus. Moreover, some patients with lymphoma may subsequently develop autoimmune abnormalities, including arthritis, and various antibodies.

This final example serves to emphasize the close links between cancer and autoimmune diseases. The function of the immune system is to keep out or destroy foreign invaders, a process that depends upon the ability to distinguish self from non-self. In addition, however, the immune system must police its own cells to make sure they are not 'turning' malignant. Any imbalance in these two roles – the immune response and the steady state regulation of cell growth and death – can lead to disease.

The genetics of autoimmunity

The immense importance of the genes—our individual blueprints—cannot be doubted: the scope and influence of the 46 pairs of human chromosomes is quite remarkable.

Population and family studies

The genetic element of autoimmunity can be analysed by population studies, family studies, and twin studies. Population studies may be misleading when analysing the frequency with which a different disease occurs in a certain area because there may well be important environmental factors that may be difficult to take out of the analysis. An example of this is the frequency with which ankylosing spondylitis (not a true autoimmune disease, but one leading to severe stiffness in the spine) is found among the Haida and Pima Native North American tribes. Because these tribes have a strikingly high frequency of a particular human leucocyte antigen (HLA B27), it was assumed that this genetic marker must be critical to the development of the disease. However, the frequent exposure of these tribes to common environmental pathogens which may trigger ankylosing spondylitis, could also be critical. These two features—genetic and environmental—are likely to be closely entwined.

With these caveats in mind, the propensity for certain ethnic groups to develop particular diseases is striking. For example, as mentioned in Chapter 1, black females in the West Indies and the United States are approximately eight times more likely to develop systemic lupus erythematosus than their Caucasian counterparts. In contrast, rheumatoid arthritis seems much more common among Caucasians in Europe than among the black, rural, population in Africa. Enthusiasm for rheumatoid arthritis being a genetically mediated disease is mitigated by the fact that urban blacks in South Africa have a much higher rate of the disease. This observation suggests strongly that environmental factors influence the development of the disease.

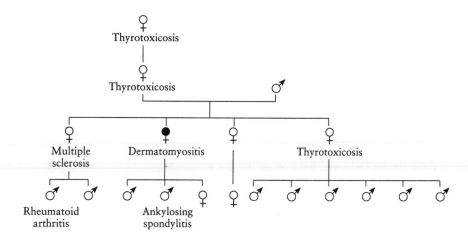

Figure 3.3 Autoimmune disease—a family history.
♀ = female; ♂ = male; ● = presenting patient.

Family studies, including studies of twins, of the development of clinical disease or the identification of autoantibodies have been very revealing. There is a well-established tendency for autoimmune diseases to run in families (see Figure 3.3). Different types of autoimmune diseases may occur in family members; a fact that supports the idea that, by small rearrangements of the factors that cause autoimmune diseases, new patterns can emerge.

Detailed analyses of multiple sclerosis occurring within families have been reported. A large population base survey from British Columbia has shown that if one member of a family has the disease, the chance of a brother or sister (sibling) developing it are 4 in 100 (4 per cent), a parent has a 3 per cent risk of developing the disease, and a child a 2.5 per cent risk. Given that the lifetime risk of somebody in that part of the world getting multiple sclerosis is approximately 0.1 per cent (1 in 1000), this represents a considerably increased risk.

Similarly, in patients with systemic lupus erythematosus, the chance of a sibling, particularly a sister, developing the disease has been estimated at approximately 2 to 3 per cent. However, it is almost unheard of for lupus to pass from a mother to her child. A very rare form of male lupus has been described in which grandfather, father, and son develop the disease.

Although much less common, scleroderma has also been reported to occur within families. There are thus a few reports describing families with two or more relatives with the disease or a closely related disorder.

Twin studies

Studies of twins—both identical and dissimilar—contribute greatly to our understanding of hereditary factors in the cause of autoimmune diseases. Since the first report of lupus in identical twins, many other cases have been described and it was estimated that if one of a pair of identical twins develops lupus there is up to a 70 per cent chance that the other twin will develop it. More recent studies suggest the true figure is under 30 per cent. In contrast, among dissimilar twins, if one of the pair develops the disease the chance that the other will do so is 5–15 per cent.

Studies of this type among patients with multiple sclerosis have not been as clear-cut, but a recent estimate suggested that, of 195 pairs of identical twins, 23 per cent were concordant (i.e. both developed the disease) for the disease, compared with 11 per cent of 280 dissimilar pairs of twins.

In a study of identical twins at King's College Hospital, London, the concordance rate for insulin-dependent diabetes was approximately 50 per cent. This is a much higher figure than that recorded for non-identical twins.

Even if the family members of patients with autoimmune diseases do not themselves develop the clinical features of the disease, many studies have shown that autoantibodies (antibodies that can bind to some part of the body's own tissues) may be present in their blood. The best examples of this have been studies of relatives of patients with systemic lupus erythematosus. Between 20 and 30 per cent of the healthy relatives of these patients have antibodies to their own DNA (especially a form called single stranded DNA). In addition these relatives have a higher incidence of positive antinuclear antibody tests (in this test antibodies to different parts of the cell nucleus are measured) as well as abnormal levels of antibodies to a range of different proteins than in the normal population. Similarly, the healthy family members of patients with autoimmune thyroid disease have been found to have anti-thyroid antibodies detectable in their serum.

These observations confirm that autoimmune phenomena, if not the diseases themselves, are not only much more common among the relatives of patients with autoimmune diseases but also make the point that the development of B cells that produce autoantibodies will not, by itself, be sufficient to cause the onset of clinical symptoms of the disease.

Autoimmune disease and the major histocompatibility complex

The term 'histocompatibility antigens' was first used to describe those antigens involved in the rejection of tissues grafted from one mouse into another mouse. The human counterpart was also first studied in the context of organ transplantation. The major histocompatibility complex (MHC; also known as the human leucocyte antigens (HLA) because they are usually found on the surface of human white blood cells) was described in Chapter 2 (see page 19). The human leucocyte antigens enable the body's immune system to recognize its own tissues, to help identify and eventually destroy foreign micro-organisms, and to control the links between mother and fetus during pregnancy. It has become clear that there is a relationship between the presence of certain types of major histocompatibility antigen types and an increased risk of autoimmune diseases.

There are three main groups of human leucocyte antigens. The genes that encode the antigens that make up these three classes in humans are found in close proximity on one particular chromosome. Unrelated individuals show considerable variation in the combinations of human leucocyte antigens on the surface of the cells of the body. An important characteristic of the human leucocyte antigens is that certain of them appear to be linked to one another—thus certain sets of these antigens seem to be inherited together.

The full range of components of the major histocompatibility antigen system is still being worked out, but it is clear that, from the moment of conception, individuals are at a greater or lesser risk of developing autoimmune diseases depending upon the combination of human leucocyte antigens on the surface of their cells.

Precisely why the genes that encode for the human leucocyte antigens predispose the individual to autoimmune diseases remains a matter of conjecture. Some of the antigens are associated with a variety of diseases, in particular HLA B8 and DR3. However it is important to remember that most individuals who express DR3 antigens on their cell surfaces are healthy. It is thought that DR3-positive individuals show a stronger and more rapid antibody response to various challenges, but tend to be low responders in a number of tests in which T cells and a variety of so-called 'accessory' cells interact. The implication of this finding is that the immune system may be less able to rid the body of potentially harmful invaders.

In certain ethnic groups there is a strong link between DR4 and rheumatoid arthritis. Furthermore, various types of DR4, which have varying susceptibility for rheumatoid arthritis in different ethnic groups, have been identified. Curiously, drug-induced lupus (notably that induced by hydralazine, a drug used to treat high blood pressure) is also related to DR4, unlike the naturally occurring form of lupus, which is more closely linked to DR3.

The complement system

The complement system has an important role in the defence of the body against infectious agents. Activation of this system is an integral part of the inflammatory process. The genes that encode for the complement components are closely linked to the class I and class II human leucocyte antigens. There are a number of genetically determined deficiencies of the complement components, two of which are worthy of particular note.

C2 deficiency

C2 deficiency is the most common complement deficiency, and the majority of patients with this condition are prone to develop a lupus-like disease, albeit with some atypical skin rashes.

C4 deficiency

It has been established that the complement C4 factor is linked to the genes that encode HLA D3. It has been suggested that the absence of a gene for one of the C4 components (there are two of these — C4A and C4B) may well be more important to the development of systemic lupus erythematosus than the presence of DR3 alone.

Hormonal aspects

A hormone is a small molecule that is released into the bloodstream from one of a number of glands and which travels in the bloodstream to a distant site where it acts. There are a large number of hormones in the body; they regulate the ways in which cells and tissues interact, grow, and reproduce.

Sex hormones

For many years it has been accepted that, under normal circumstances, the immune system in women differs from that in men because:

- Women are generally more resistant to infections. Their longer life expectancy may be due, in part, to this fact.
- Women have a higher serum level of immunoglobulins G and M, which may be linked to their ability to resist infections.

- The female immune system is generally able to react more powerfully when stimulated.

However, the other side of the coin is that most diseases of the immune system are much more common in women than men. This is most obvious in systemic lupus erythematosus, where the ratio of female to male patients is 10 to 1, followed closely by scleroderma and Sjögren's syndrome (9 to 1) and Graves' disease associated with an overactive thyroid gland, where the ratio of affected females to males is 7 to 1.

Men and women are exposed to different hormonal influences, although, in fact, they produce both 'male' and 'female' sex hormones—no sex hormones are unique to either sex. What differentiates the sexes is the different levels of particular sex hormones; males having relatively high concentrations of androgens and females having relatively high levels of oestrogen and progesterone.

Hormone levels fluctuate markedly during life, most notably during adolescence, pregnancy, and the period of time immediately following childbirth. This period in particular seems to be associated with the start of several autoimmune diseases. Immediately the placenta is ejected there is a drastic decrease in the oestrogen levels, and an even larger fall in progesterone levels. There is also little doubt that oral contraceptives, especially those with moderate or high doses of oestrogen, can exacerbate or even induce a relapse of quiescent autoimmune disease. Healthy women with no clinical signs or symptoms of autoimmunity have been reported to develop features similar to those of rheumatoid arthritis while using the contraceptive pill. However, several studies have indicated that the pill either protects against or postpones the development of severe rheumatoid arthritis, although the reason is unknown.

The way in which sex hormones are metabolized by the body has been examined in some detail in patients with systemic lupus erythematosus. There are some reports of high oestrogen levels in both females and males with this disease. Male patients with lupus have also been shown to have lower levels of the male sex hormone testosterone.

Further evidence of a hormonal link with systemic lupus erythematosus comes from genetic analysis of a curious condition known as Kleinefelter's syndrome. Sufferers appear to be male but have a reduced sperm count, little development of the testes, and some breast development. Analysis of their chromosomes has shown that, although male, they have an extra X chromosome and that this is responsible for their unusual appearance. The condition is associated with an increased risk of systemic lupus erythematosus.

Animal studies

Many animal studies have investigated the effects of sex hormones in mouse models of lupus. The main observations can be summarized as follows:

- Female animals develop lupus-like disease earlier and die younger than their male counterparts.
- Administration of oestrogen to males greatly increases their mortality rate compared with males treated with male sex hormones.
- Oestrogen treatment of males accelerates the kidney disease, while treatment with male sex hormones (androgens) appears to prevent this problem.
- Castration of males before reaching sexual maturity accelerates the rate of development of disease and hastens death.
- Androgen treatment of females slows the progress of disease.

Similar studies have been undertaken in a rat model of autoimmune thyroid disease with rather similar results:

- Castration of males leads to the appearance of autoimmune thyroiditis, which is identical in both incidence and severity to that seen in female rats.
- Administration of testosterone to castrated males and to normal females leads to clinical improvement. The degree of improvement is related to the dose of the hormone.
- Treatment with testosterone is beneficial to these animals, sometimes leading to a complete regression of the disease.

Pregnancy

Pregnancy has major effects on many of the autoimmune diseases and affects different diseases in different ways, for example:

- Rheumatoid arthritis—most patients with rheumatoid arthritis improve during pregnancy but the disease almost always flares up again after the birth of the child.
- Systemic lupus erythematosus—some patients find that their disease becomes much more active during pregnancy but in most cases SLE in pregnancy is more of a threat to the fetus than to the mother.

Thus the effect of the hormones is simply one of the factors that determine the type of autoimmune disease a patient will develop and how active it will be.

The thymus and autoimmunity

The thymus secretes a family of hormone-like substances called thymic hormones. These play a central role in organizing and controlling immune reactions through the way in which they help T cells to differentiate into helper or suppressor/cytotoxic cells.

It is only in the last 30 years that the important physiological role of the thymus in the early development of the immune system has been established. Its importance was confirmed when the removal of the gland very early in life in experimental animals resulted in a marked, progressive loss of immune functions, causing death due to infections. It was later shown that implantation of thymus tissue led to partial or complete restoration of immune function.

Animal studies

These early observations prompted examination of the role of the thymus in autoimmunity:

- In the New Zealand black/white mouse (an animal model of lupus), the thymus atrophies (shrivels up) early in life.
- The removal of the thymus from normal mice very early in life is followed by the appearance of autoantibodies by 8 weeks of age.
- Removal of the thymus of adult mice is associated with autoimmune phenomena.
- Removal of the thymus in animals prone to autoimmunity has been shown to accelerate the autoimmunity.
- Thymus transplantation in these animals corrects some of the immune defects.
- Thymic hormones have been shown to have a regulating effect in various models of autoimmune thyroiditis and multiple sclerosis.

An interesting link between the thymus and diet in the New Zealand black mouse (which also develops a form of lupus) was established when it was shown that low-calorie diets delay thymic atrophy and the emergence of immune defects, thus prolonging survival.

Human studies

Studies in patients have generally been less rewarding than animal studies. Abnormalities of the thymus are rarely present in patients with auto-immune diseases. Many people who develop myasthenia gravis as adults have an enlarged thymus, and the disease is often improved by removal of the gland. In addition, the coexistence of lupus and myasthenia gravis is more common than might be expected. Furthermore, lupus has been known to develop after thymectomy (removal of thymus) for myasthenia gravis.

The reason why removal of the thymus might help patients with myasthenia gravis, which is characterized by muscular weakness, is not entirely clear. It is generally accepted that thymic hormones accelerate the maturation of T helper cells, which are known to bind to the receptors on the muscle cells that receive stimulation from the nervous system. It may be that in myasthenia gravis there are too many T helper cells in the tissues, that they block nerve stimulation of the muscle, and that by removing the gland a reduction in these cells is achieved, thus allowing more normal activation of muscle contraction.

Sex hormones and thymic hormones

It is important to remember that the factors that are described here do not operate in isolation. A good example of this is the interesting interaction that occurs between sex and thymic hormones. Injections of one form of oestrogen have been shown to decrease the size of the thymus and to cause a reduction in the level of thymic hormone in the blood. Furthermore, it has been shown that the level of thymic hormone is markedly decreased in the blood of women who are either post-menopausal or who have had their ovaries removed and are undergoing oestrogen therapy.

In experiments in a mouse model of lupus, the effects of long-term administration of testosterone and a thymic hormone known as thymosine were studied. Thymosine treatment that had been started in castrated animals and continued through life abolished the rise in anti-DNA antibodies. This observation suggests that, in these mice, androgens work throughout the first months of life to suppress the production of anti-DNA antibodies. Indeed it was also shown that lack of these androgens, even for a relatively brief period, allowed anti-DNA antibody production to begin. Once initiated, this process proved very difficult to suppress.

Steroids

Although steroids are often thought of as drugs given for the treatment of a wide range of diseases, they are in fact produced naturally by the adrenal glands (which are situated adjacent to the kidneys) and are also called corticosteroids.

Action

Corticosteroids have a wide variety of effects in the body. Their main actions are brought about by their diffusing through the cell membrane to bind to a receptor protein in the cytoplasm and form a complex. This complex enters the cell nucleus and can affect protein manufacture. Thus corticosteroids can increase the production of different proteins in different tissues—the majority of proteins produced by the actions of corticosteroids are enzymes.

Corticosteroids can have anti-inflammatory effects. They can reduce the flow of blood in small veins or capillaries, thus stopping white blood cells from passing towards a site of inflammation. They can also impair the ability of white blood cells (especially the neutrophils) to destroy cells and kill bacteria. They have many other effects, including:

- reducing the numbers of lymphocytes;
- inhibiting the release of the chemical messenger histamine (which is often involved in inflammation);
- altering the actions of the complement system.

As well as these functions, corticosteroids also have marked effects on the immune system helping to reduce inflammation as follows:

- They cause an increase in the numbers of neutrophils, probably by encouraging their release from the bone marrow.
- They impair the ability of neutrophils to stick to the lining cells of the blood vessels and pass into the tissues.
- They reduce the numbers of circulating T suppressor cells, monocytes, eosinophils, and basophils.
- They reduce the production of antibodies by the B cells.
- They destroy some T cells.
- They reduce the macrophage response to antigens.

Although the body is capable of producing modest quantities of corticosteroids, it has now been clearly established that synthetic forms of these drugs can have major beneficial effects in a wide range of autoimmune diseases. Unfortunately, on occasion the benefits may be outweighed by their side-effects (see page 110).

Diet

Diet is another piece of the jigsaw of autoimmunity. Almost every part of the diet including total calories, fats, protein, minerals, and vitamins, has now been analysed to see if an excess or restriction of any individual component, or combination of components, can affect the way the immune system works.

Calorie restriction

During the siege of Paris in the Franco-Prussian war of 1870, a French physician noted that enforced starvation of many of his patients with diabetes seemed to help relieve some of the symptoms of this condition. Because of the obvious problems with patient compliance, this approach to the treatment of autoimmune disease has been relatively little studied in man, although a report has suggested that reduction in total calories can improve some of the symptoms of rheumatoid arthritis. However, there have been several studies of calorie restriction in animals with various autoimmune conditions. Thus, in one of the types of mouse that spontaneously develops a condition resembling systemic lupus erythematosus, it was shown that reduction in the total amount of calories seemed to protect the animals against inflammation in the kidneys, and helped to increase their lifespan. In another study, it was suggested that the way this approach worked was to reduce the levels of immune complexes circulating in the blood and deposition of immunoglobulins and complement in the kidneys of a lupus mouse model.

Amino acid restriction

A restricted amino acid diet has been shown to prolong survival and prevent the inflammation in one of the lupus-prone types of mouse model. Other studies have suggested that a synthetic amino acid diet can also prolong survival and reduce antibody levels. In contrast, monkeys fed diets high in alfalfa seeds have developed abnormalities in blood tests rather similar to human lupus. This effect has been attributed to a particular amino acid that is present in high concentration in alfalfa seeds and sprouts. More recently, a similar reaction has been suspected in human subjects.

Dietary fat restriction

The influence of dietary fat on autoimmunity in mice appears to be particularly important. It has been shown that diets relatively high in fat have increased production of autoantibodies and abnormalities in lymphocyte function. In contrast it has been reported that low fat diets can reduce kidney inflammation and autoantibody levels as well as prolonging the life span of lupus-prone animals.

The precise nature of the fat used in these experiments appears to be important. It seems that diets enriched with certain fish oils can protect female mice from developing kidney inflammation. The effect of fat on autoimmunity is very probably derived from its action on the synthesis of the chemical messengers prostaglandins and leucotrienes. In more recent studies, patients with rheumatoid arthritis and lupus have been given a low fat diet supplemented by various fish oils. Although there has been no uniform agreement as to how successful these studies have been, the obvious advantages of 'culinary compromise' compared with drug therapy make this a very attractive option. Even a small reduction in the requirement for steroids or other powerful drugs must be considered beneficial.

Mineral deficiency

The influence of certain minerals, in particular zinc and selenium, has also been studied in animals. Thus, lupus-prone mice put on to a diet that was deliberately low in zinc were found to have a decreased rate of self-destruction of the red blood cells, which causes anaemia and kidney inflammation. Keeping the animals on zinc-deficient diets was also associated with lower levels of autoantibodies and a prolonged lifespan. Selenium supplementation of the diet was also shown to improve the survival in one type of lupus-prone mouse.

Vitamin deficiency

Vitamin A
A diet deficient in vitamin A aggravates autoimmunity in one lupus-prone type of mouse.

Vitamin C
Intriguing, and quite unexplained, is the claim that vitamin C protects guinea pigs from a characteristic inflammation of the brain tissues that mimics multiple sclerosis.

Vitamin D
There is increasing evidence this vitamin is intimately involved in the normal functioning of the immune system. Its main function is to control the level of calcium in the blood. Too low a calcium level is associated with muscular spasms, a tingling sensation around the mouth and in the limbs, and a feeling of generalized weakness; too high a level may lead to calcium being deposited in soft tissues of the body and, in severe cases, to generalized collapse, which may mimic the symptoms of a heart attack. To undertake its role as the calcium 'policeman', vitamin D works very closely with a hormone—parathormone—which is released by the para-

thyroid glands (four small glands situated immediately behind the thyroid gland in the neck). These two compounds control the uptake of calcium from the diet, its resorption from bone, and its excretion into the urine.

Of great interest to immunologists, vitamin D has been shown to inhibit the production of antibodies by B cells. It can also inhibit the production of the chemical messenger, interleukin-2, and may also stop T cells from multiplying. It also seems likely that vitamin D3 has an effect on the human leucocyte antigen molecules that appear on the surfaces of most types of cells. These actions imply that normal production and function of vitamin D is an important component of the immune system, and that abnormalities in vitamin D production may predispose to abnormalities in immune function, including the development of autoimmunity.

Vitamin D also affects the way white blood cells develop, increases the ability of white cells (notably macrophages) to kill bacteria, and increases the production of various chemical messengers (notably tumour necrosis factor) from white cells in the peripheral blood. It can also induce these white blood cells to produce a special variety of proteins, known as heat shock proteins (see page 33), which may be involved in auto-immunity.

Although concentrations in the blood of the two types of vitamin D referred to above have been found to be normal in patients with rheumatoid arthritis, the level of 1,25(dihydroxy) vitamin D3 is significantly lower in patients with overactive thyroid disease and insulin-dependent diabetes.

The effects of vitamin D on autoimmune disease in a lupus-prone strain of mouse have also been described. Although the hormone did not appear to alter antibody production, the amount of protein escaping into the urine of the mouse was significantly reduced. Active vitamin D3 appears able to regulate the expansion of activated T cells.

Vitamin E
It has been shown that a vitamin E enriched diet will prolong survival and it has been claimed that patients with lupus, scleroderma, and polymyositis improved when their diets were supplemented with vitamin E.

Ageing

It has become increasingly evident that just as getting older is associated with the skin becoming wrinkled and the hair becoming thin and grey, so there is a gradual decay in the efficient functioning of the immune system. This process has been studied in both animals and people.

Autoantibodies

Perhaps the best studied aspect of immunological decay is the increased presence of autoantibodies detectable in the blood of elderly individuals. However, it should be emphasized that autoimmune diseases are not characteristic of old age. This may be because other factors, notably the hormonal balance, have changed, which may outweigh any untoward effects of the ageing process on the immune system. However, there does seem to be a steady rise in the prevalence of a wide variety of auto-antibodies with age.

Rheumatoid factor (see page 72) was the first autoantibody whose frequency was reported to increase with age—its prevalence in elderly subjects ranges from 19 to 42 per cent, compared with 2 per cent or less in young individuals. Similarly the frequency of antinuclear antibodies is significantly higher in elderly people (10 to 37 per cent) than in the young (0 to 6 per cent).

Abnormal responses

Abnormal responses by immune cells to various challenges at different times in the lifespan have been examined and several age-related changes have been found. The net result of these changes is a gradual decline, with age, in the ability of the immune system to defend the body against infection and to prevent the development of cancer. In general there seems to be:

- a decrease in the number of both T helper and T suppressor/cytotoxic cells;
- a progressive decline in the ability of lymphocytes to respond to certain forms of stimulation. This effect seems to get progressively worse from birth;
- a reduction in the number of chemical messengers released by the T cells;
- a reduction in the production of receptors on T cells to receive chemical messengers.

Not all researchers agree that these defects occur with age. Some authors have found little change in the numbers of T cells, but it does seem widely accepted that T cell functions decline with age, although, confusingly, some groups have reported an apparent increase in T helper cell function in the elderly. A Japanese group has suggested that there might be a selection process going on in the elderly whereby functioning of the immune system in those individuals who survive to the age of 90 and beyond is notably maintained. These individuals seem to have the least decrease in immune responses tested.

Antibody abnormalities

That age appears to have many different effects is also emphasized by studies of the way in which sugar molecules are attached to a particular immunoglobulin—immunoglobulin G (IgG).

An increase in the number of immunoglobulin molecules with a reduced level of a particular type of attached sugar molecule (galactose) is a feature of rheumatoid arthritis. However, the interpretation of the levels of IgG with a reduced sugar content depends upon the age of the patient, as sugar levels vary with age:

- At birth, most IgG molecules have a full set of sugars attached.
- By 1 year of age, approximately 50 per cent of the IgG molecules of healthy children have a reduced sugar content.
- Between the ages of 1 and 15 this figure falls back to between 15 and 20 per cent, and remains constant until around the age of 40.
- After 40, there is a steady rise in the number of immunoglobulins that lack sugar.
- By the age of 80, even healthy people have close to 60 per cent of immunoglobulin molecules with a reduced amount of sugar.

Thus, in patients with rheumatoid arthritis allowance has to be made for the patient's age to be sure that the levels of IgG with low galactose levels are really abnormal.

Drugs

It is perhaps more than a little ironic that many of the drugs used for therapeutic purposes can also, on occasion, induce autoimmunity. Some drugs can produce conditions that mimic individual autoimmune diseases while others have more diverse effects. No drug alone can cause an autoimmune condition unless other factors, such as human leucocyte antigen type, hormonal imbalances, etc., are also present.

It is evident that a variety of drugs can, under certain circumstances, induce conditions that mimic naturally occurring autoimmune diseases. Among these drugs it is evident that 6D-penicillamine occupies pride of place. No less than seven different autoimmune diseases are known to occur occasionally following therapy with this drug:

- lupus erythematosus;
- myasthenia gravis;
- myositis;
- haemolytic anaemia;
- thrombocytopenia;
- pemphigus;
- scleroderma.

Drug-induced lupus

Although there are similarities between 'naturally occurring' lupus and the condition caused by certain drugs, there are also a number of important differences. In essence, while joint pain and skin rashes occur in both types of lupus, disease of the kidney and brain, which are common in the naturally occurring condition, are rare in drug-induced disease. For lupus to be clearly drug-induced, there must be a history of the signs and symptoms developing after a drug has been prescribed, followed by an appropriate remission of symptoms when drug treatment is stopped. A recurrence of the symptoms on re-exposure to the drug is confirmation of the association; however, in clinical practice this should (we hope!) be a rare event.

Drug-induced lupus was first described in 1945. Since then many drugs have been incriminated. It is now known that drugs with a variety of different molecular structures can cause lupus; several of these drugs are used for treating high blood pressure. For this reason, drug-induced lupus tends to occur more often in older individuals than the 'natural' form. Furthermore, approximately equal numbers of men and women develop drug-induced lupus, quite unlike the 'natural' disease, in which females predominate; there are very few reports of drug-related lupus among the Afro-Caribbean population.

It appears that a substantial amount of the drug has to be taken before the lupus-like symptoms appear. In practice, this often means patients will be on the drug for 1 to 2 years before the joint pains and/or skin rash start. It may therefore be a while before the patient or physician realizes that it is the drug that is responsible.

It has been shown that individuals with a genetic tendency to metabolize drugs slowly are most likely to develop the condition. An interaction between human leucocyte antigen type and drug-induced lupus has been described with patients who are prescribed hydralazine for high blood pressure. It has also been shown than those individuals who carry the DR4 class II human leucocyte antigen (see page 19) are much more likely to develop lupus-like disease.

Some individuals do not develop the clinical features of lupus but do have detectable antinuclear antibodies. Indeed, it has been estimated that up to a quarter of individuals treated for high blood pressure with hydralazine will develop antinuclear antibodies, which are virtually always present in individuals showing symptoms of the disease.

Not surprisingly, therapy for drug-induced lupus consists first in recognizing that it is the drug that is responsible and then stopping it. For most patients this is sufficient and the symptoms resolve within days or weeks. Occasionally symptoms may persist for several months and, occasionally, involvement of the heart or lungs has required treatment with corticosteroids.

Drug-induced myasthenia gravis

In the mid-1970s a number of patients with rheumatoid arthritis developed myasthenia gravis (see page 95) while taking the drug D-penicillamine for their arthritis. As myasthenia gravis very rarely complicates rheumatoid arthritis, its onset in these patients shortly after starting D-penicillamine suggested that the drug might have precipitated the condition. Later the characteristic autoantibodies associated with myasthenia gravis were shown to be present in a number of the rheumatoid arthritis patients who had received D-penicillamine treatment for several months.

Subsequently, it has been suggested that approximately 1 per cent of rheumatoid arthritis patients treated with D-penicillamine will develop myasthenia gravis or something like it. The duration of penicillamine therapy before the onset of myasthenia gravis has been reported to vary enormously from 2 days to 5 years, with an average of 8 months. There has not, however, been any really good evidence of a relationship between the cumulative dosage and severity of the symptoms. In general the symptoms and signs of myasthenia disappear completely with withdrawal of the drug.

Several other drugs have been incriminated in drug-induced myasthenia gravis. These include trimethadone and diphenylhydantoin, both used in the treatment of epilepsy. Occasionally myasthenia gravis has been associated with quinidine and propanolol (used in the treatment of irregular heartbeat), and with lithium (used in patients with mania). It should be emphasized that this is a rare complication with these drugs.

Drug-induced myositis

It has been established that a number of drugs are directly toxic to muscle but that a true drug-induced inflammatory condition is most unusual. However, such a condition has been associated with D-penicillamine, penicillin, sulphonamides, procainamide, hydralazine, and tamoxifen (a drug used in the treatment of breast cancer).

It has been estimated that up to 1 per cent of patients treated with D-penicillamine may also develop myositis (see page 97). Patients with D-penicillamine-induced myositis seem particularly likely to develop swallowing difficulties and severe muscle weakness. Drug-induced myositis can be fatal.

Drug-induced haemolytic anaemia

Over 20 per cent of cases of haemolytic anaemia (see page 98) previously thought to be of unknown cause are now thought to be caused by pharmaceutical products. The destruction of red blood cells is caused by antibodies that bind to these cells, which have in some way been altered by the offending drug. The frequency of these so-called haemolytic anaemias seems to be rising.

There are various explanations as to why or how drugs might affect red blood cells. They could bind to the surface of the red cells and thus fool the immune system into thinking that the membrane of the red cells is some 'foreign' material. Alternatively the drugs might stimulate the B cells to produce antibodies that bind to the surface of the red cell.

Many drugs have been associated with haemolytic anaemia. Of these, methyldopa (used to treat high blood pressure), the penicillins, quinine, and quinadine are the best known. Methyldopa-induced haemolytic anaemia has been researched most. It appears to develop 4 to 6 months after treatment, but occasionally the onset has been delayed by 1 or 2 years. If it is not recognized in time this condition may become severe and even life-threatening.

Drug-induced thrombocytopenia (low platelet count)

Over 50 different medications are known to induce thrombocytopenia (see page 98). As these cells are critical to the ability of the blood to clot, their destruction has serious consequences.

The best known offenders are the gold salts (used in the treatment of rheumatoid arthritis), heparin (used to treat thrombosis), and the cinchona alkaloids (which are used in the treatment of various cancers). D-penicillamine may also, on occasion, give rise to thrombocytopenia.

Drug-induced pemphigus

Pemphigus is a severe disease of the skin that is characterized by blister formation in the outer layers (see page 99). The naturally occurring disease is rare but drug-induced forms have been associated with D-penicillamine and captopril (a drug used to lower blood pressure). The pathology of penicillamine-induced pemphigus is indistinguishable from the naturally occurring form and its course is variable. Although the majority of patients are disease-free within 4 months of stopping the drug, other unfortunate individuals continue to suffer the severe blisters for many months.

Drug-induced scleroderma

Scleroderma, which causes increased thickening of the skin and of some internal tissues (see page 87), may be induced by a number of drugs, in particular bleomycin (an antitumour drug), D-penicillamine, pentazocine (used for pain relief), and appetite suppressants. As with the other drug-induced conditions, cessation of drug therapy is essential to prevent further progression of the disease.

Toxins and chemicals

Smoking

Given the now well-established links between smoking and cancer (especially lung cancer) and various chronic inflammatory diseases (such as chronic bronchitis) many attempts have been made to study the effects of cigarette smoke on the immune system.

These endeavours have not been helped by the fact that smoke is made up of many components and almost certainly has different effects in different parts of the respiratory system. However, various deleterious effects of smoke on the immune system have been claimed, including an increase in the total level of immunoglobulin E (IgE) in the blood and a reduction in the amount of IgA, and an accompanying increase in the IgM level, in saliva. These alterations in immunoglobulin production from the lining cells of the upper respiratory tract are probably important as a marker of underlying changes in the function of the immune system. It has been shown that the lining of the upper and lower parts of the respiratory tract of smokers have reduced numbers of an important group of cells known as the Langerhans' cells. It has further been suggested that this smoking-related reduction of Langerhans' cells might predispose to viral infection and to an inadequate response to malignant change. However, it must be said that at the present time the precise link between these types of change and smoking remains uncertain.

The effects of smoking on autoimmune diseases have not been studied extensively, although some work has been done on patients suffering from Goodpasture's syndrome (a condition in which antibodies are formed against cells in the kidney and lungs). It has been shown that most of the patients with Goodpasture's syndrome who smoke tend to suffer from severe bleeding in the lungs; a complication rare in those who do not smoke.

Silicon and silicates

Silicon implants (used in breast enlargement operations) have been reported to cause a variety of symptoms, including joint pain and swelling, and conditions resembling lupus and scleroderma. Indeed, at the time of writing (January 1994) the United States Food and Drug Administration has expressed grave concern about the safety of breast enlargement surgery and has recommended that such operations cease until the implants can be demonstrated to be leakproof or until an alternative filler material can be found. However, most experts are not convinced that their implants cause disease.

A clear link has also been established between exposure of gold miners in South Africa to silicates and scleroderma.

Spanish oil syndrome

During the 1980s in Spain over 20,000 people were affected by a condition that came to be known as 'the Spanish oil syndrome'. This was caused by the deliberate contamination of rape seed oil, which was used for cooking. The illness had two phases:

- Phase 1—fever, rash, abdominal upset, and symptoms that suggested inflammation of the nervous system.
- Phase 2—the development of Raynaud's phenomenon, hardening of the skin, hair loss, dryness of the mouth, arthritis, and contracture of certain joints.

In its latter stages, the condition resembles scleroderma. It is thought that over 300 people died from this syndrome.

Plastics and solvents

Thickening of the skin, similar to that seen in scleroderma, has been shown to follow exposure to polyvinyl chloride (PVC). Although patients presenting with this problem have a number of clinical features suggestive of scleroderma, they do not have any of the autoantibodies that are characteristic of the disease. They do, however, show a common predisposition to a certain human leucocyte antigen type (HLA DR5).

Exposure to various other plastics and solvents, including epoxy resins, methane, trichlorethylene, benzene, and xylene, has been associated with skin changes resembling scleroderma. Likewise, exposure to paraphenylene diamine, which was once used in hair dyes, results in a variety of features typical of the autoimmune diseases, including rheumatoid nodules and a type of skin necrosis.

Sunlight

Sunlight is an environmental hazard. A particular wavelength of sunlight —ultraviolet (UV) light—is a type of radiation and a serious health hazard.

At the time of their initial diagnosis, many patients with systemic lupus erythematosus (and particularly those presenting with skin rash), can recall recent exposure to strong and/or prolonged sunlight. Because the link between lupus and ultraviolet light is now unequivocal, it is standard clinical practice for doctors to recommend that their patients protect themselves from ultraviolet exposure. A worrying development in this area is the destruction of the ozone layer by chlorofluorocarbons (CFCs), the chemicals found in refrigeration systems and aerosol cans. Holes in the ozone layer, which shields the earth from UV irradiation, are increasing in size and threaten an increase in the number of cases of malignant melanoma (a form of skin cancer). Malignant melanoma has reached epidemic proportions over the last decade due to the predilection of Caucasians for spending their summer holidays acquiring a sun tan. No one has yet estimated the increase of lupus during the same period, but it may have increased at the same rate as other skin-associated, ultraviolet-induced diseases. The Canadian government recently took the unusual step of warning its citizens not to go out in the sun without adequate protection.

Stress

The term 'stress' is rather vague and means different things to different people. It has thus been difficult to establish a direct correlation between even major stressful life events, such as marriage, bereavement, or examinations, and the initiation or exacerbation of autoimmune disease. However, most clinicians meet patients in whom the association between stress and disease does seem clear. Thus, despite the rather intangible nature of 'stress' it may well be that this is one of the various environmental factors involved in stimulating autoimmune disease.

Among some of the better established correlations, it has been shown that the onset of insulin-dependent diabetes, which occurs mainly in children, may be associated with stress. Thus the death of a parent or the separation or divorce of the parents, have been shown to correlate with the onset of autoimmune disease. These data do not suggest that the affected child would never have developed the disease had these particular life events not occurred, merely that there may be a link with the time of onset in the given individual. Similarly, it has been shown that a recurrence of uveitis (inflammation in certain tissues of the eye) has been linked to divorce, business losses, and examination failure; the onset of Crohn's disease has been associated with bereavement, pregnancy, marriage or divorce, and moving house; finally, the onset and severity of rheumatoid arthritis has also be shown to be associated with stress. Women patients with rheumatoid arthritis are on the whole more nervous, tense, worried, and moody than their healthy female siblings.

However, these sorts of reports must not be taken at face value, as they could reflect secondary psychological responses to a primary physical disease. It has been shown that those patients unable to cope emotionally with their disease appear to be more likely to have a rapid and progressive disability, having responded poorly to treatment.

It must be emphasized that it can be difficult to distinguish 'pure stress' from other factors, such as diet, which can also affect the immune system. For example, studies on the effect of stress in rheumatoid arthritis must take account of the fact that the swollen painful hands greatly restrict the type of food that the patient can prepare and eat. Similarly, involvement of the jaw joints can restrict the types of food eaten. As has been discussed, calorie restriction and alteration in the balance of the diet have profound effects on the immune system.

4

How do autoimmune diseases develop? The interplay of the factors

No single factor can cause an autoimmune disease: it is most likely that several interact in a variety of ways to produce such an illness. In this chapter we will look at these factors and examine the ways in which they can co-operate to produce a disease. In considering these issues we will:

- Examine, in detail, the interplay of the disease-causing factors using two analogies: the mosaic model and the card game.
- Analyse the role of T and B lymphocytes and see how an imbalance in either cell population can result in an increased risk of disease.
- Make comparisons with the yin–yang of Eastern philosophy.
- Use rheumatoid arthritis as a 'model' for autoimmunity, and place some of the immune imbalances in the context of an actual disease.

The interplay of biological factors in autoimmunity

The many factors that can influence the development of autoimmune disease were discussed in Chapter 3. This chapter will look at the ways in which these factors interact.

The mosaic analogy

A useful analogy for the background to autoimmune diseases is a mosaic. The *Concise Oxford Dictionary* defines a mosaic as 'the process of producing pictures or patterns by cementing together small pieces of stone, glass, etc.' The definition implies that, by reassembling the same pieces in a different order, another pattern or picture will emerge. Much the same process can be seen with diseases of the immune system. The 'small pieces' in this case include:

- genetic (inherited) factors;
- effects of diet and hormones;

- infections;
- abnormalities in the complement enzyme system.

By rearranging these pieces different patterns of disease are revealed (see Figure 4.1).

The idea of rearranging the pieces of a mosaic (i.e. the factors that contribute to disease) to derive a different picture (i.e. disease) also draws an analogy with the concept that the same factors might cause a variety of diseases, depending on the way they interact (intersect). In Figure 4.2

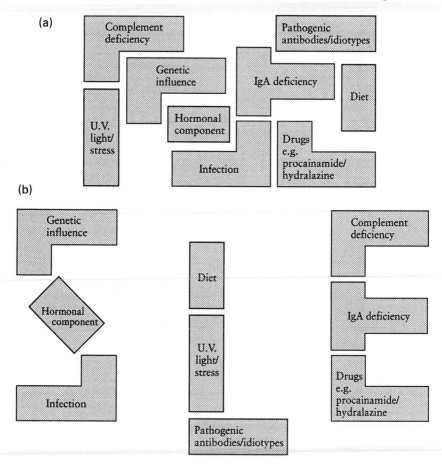

Figure 4.1 (a) The various pieces of the mosaic which show the background to developing an autoimmune disease—they are arranged as a rectangle. (b) Using exactly the same pieces but rearranging them so the letters SLE (systemic lupus erythematosus) are formed. The point that the same factors—albeit rearranged—underlie most if not all autoimmune diseases is thus emphasized.

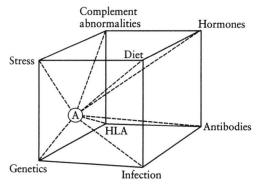

Multiple Intersect Theory - Disease A

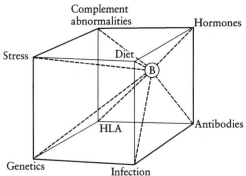

Multiple Intersect Theory - Disease B

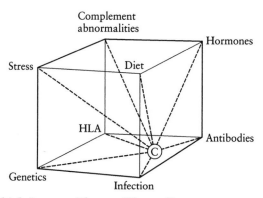

Multiple Intersect Theory - Disease C

Figure 4.2 The three-dimensional intersect model showing how lines starting from the same positions may intersect at different places (here shown as A, B, C). By analogy different autoimmune diseases may derive from much the same factors.

we have extended this analogy to a three-dimensional model, which shows that the same multiple disease factors may provide several points of intersection. This model, called the 'multiple intersect model', may be applied to real life events in which genetic, environmental, and other factors come together in different ways that determine whether the individual develops disease A, B, or C. Support for this concept comes from the fact that approximately one-third of lupus erythematosus patients have a relative with another autoimmune disease.

The card game analogy

The mosaic analogy implies that exactly the same factors are involved in the induction of every autoimmune disease. As this is unlikely to be the case, a more flexible model is needed to reflect the causes of autoimmune diseases with greater precision.

Imagine a new card game which we will call 'Health'. The cards have a variety of titles, such as 'female' (or 'male'), 'high fat diet' (or 'low fat diet'), 'infection' (with a variety of infectious organisms), 'complement deficiency', 'antibodies' (of various sorts), etc. A hand of, say, seven cards is dealt and the object of the game is to avoid certain combinations of cards that if held together constitute a 'disease'. For example, a combination of cards (Figure 4.3) marked 'high level rheumatoid factor', 'female', 'age 30 to 55', 'human leucocyte antigen DR4', 'high fat diet', 'infection with Epstein–Barr virus', and 'abnormal glycosylation of IgG' constitutes a 'rheumatoid hand'—clearly to be avoided! Another combination (Figure 4.4)

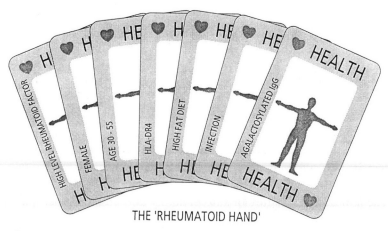

THE 'RHEUMATOID HAND'

Figure 4.3 The game of 'Health'. A hand of cards is dealt representing the different factors likely to be important in the cause of rheumatoid arthritis.

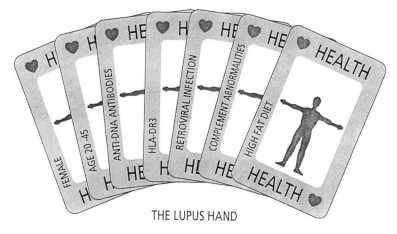

THE LUPUS HAND

Figure 4.4 The card pack has been shuffled and another hand dealt, this time representing the factors important in the development of systemic lupus erythematosus.

of 'female', 'age 20 to 45', 'with anti-DNA antibody production', 'human leucocyte antigen DR3', 'retroviral infection', 'complement abnormalities', and 'high fat diet' would make up a 'lupus hand'. Thus, by analogy, the development of an autoimmune disease requires many contributory factors to be present. As a corollary individuals may be dealt successively 'bad' hands predisposing them to more than one disease. Thus, some unfortunate people may develop lupus, Sjögren's syndrome, and an under-active thyroid gland (Hashimoto's disease).

The big picture

The mosaic and card game analogies serve to emphasize that autoimmune diseases occur only after the interaction of many factors. What remains more uncertain, and is the subject of much current medical research, is the precise interplay between these factors. These interactions are often subtle and invariably complicated. Nevertheless, we will attempt to outline a scheme for an autoimmune battlefield and then put this in the context of a specific disease.

The multifactorial nature of autoimmunity also poses another question directly relevant to treatment: how many of these factors must be corrected or reversed so that the disease can be dissipated or at least brought under control?

The B cells

'Self-reactive' autoantibodies and cytotoxic T cells are central to the damage that occurs in autoimmune disease. Consider first the B cell or, perhaps more appropriately, its antibody-producing offspring, the plasma cell. As can be seen from Figure 4.5, although a given clone of cells may be able to produce autoantibodies, whether it does or not depends on many factors. It is now evident that a certain amount of carefully controlled autoantibody production is part of the normal development of the immune system. The bulk of scientific evidence suggests that the plasma cells producing these autoantibodies are functioning correctly and, for the most part, are producing antibodies that are part of the body's normal repertoire. In an immunological war crimes trial, B cells/plasma cells might be thought of as subordinates, claiming that they were simply 'following orders' from their T cell superior officers. Nevertheless, there are circumstances in which B cells undertake independent action and are thus responsible for an autoimmune state. For example, with age the B cell population may become malignant—B cell cancers sometimes arise; those that produce antibodies are known as myelomas.

B cell cancers

When a cancerous B cell divides and multiplies in an uncontrolled fashion it produces substantial quantities of unwanted antibody, which may bind to a self-antigen. Usually, however, an 'irrelevant' antibody with no damaging autoimmune effects is manufactured, and the blood becomes thick or viscous because of the large numbers of this antibody. This can be treated relatively easily but it is now being recognized (see Chapter 3, page 27) that around a quarter of the antibodies produced by B cell myelomas can react with self proteins and are, in fact, autoantibodies.

Very high levels of unwanted antibodies can be present in the blood of patients with myeloma but, in fact, these patients rarely develop autoimmune symptoms. This observation is good evidence that antibodies alone rarely induce the symptoms and signs of an autoimmune disease.

B cell activation

B cells can also be activated after exposure to certain infections, chemicals, or even foreign blood cells (which may happen after a blood transfusion or a transplant). This phenomenon is called polyclonal activation and results in the production of many different types of unnecessary anti-

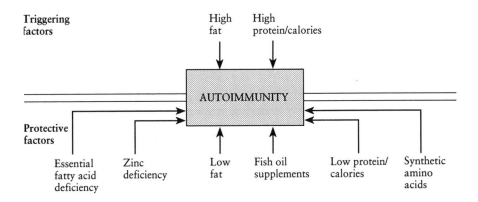

Figure 4.5 The influence of dietary fat on the immune system.

bodies, including those that can react with host tissues. As we will see later, whether or not an autoimmune disease results from such activation depends on other factors, but clearly such an event has the potential to bring about a serious autoimmune condition.

Immune complexes

Antigen–antibody immune complexes occur quite frequently and are, quite literally, complexes of the autoantibody and the tissue with which it reacts. In the case of a normal immune response, the complex will be made up of the antibody and a microbe (or part of a microbe)—this complex is part of the body's mechanism system for eliminating foreign antigens. Immune complexes can form anywhere in the body and are deposited in various tissues, including the kidney, skin, joint, and nervous system. They have certain characteristics that determine whether they become harmful and cause tissue damage:

- After deposition, complement may be activated or 'fixed' (see Chapter 3), causing damage to adjacent 'innocent' tissues.
- Granulocytes often infiltrate the tissues, attracted by fragments of the complement cascade and cause further damage by releasing enzymes that break down protein.

Although the formation of immune complexes is part of a normal immune response, sustained production can lead to inflammation and autoimmune disease.

The T cells

T cells are responsible for many tasks involved in the regulation of the immune system. As discussed in Chapter 2 they:

- process antigens;
- determine the type of immune response;
- determine the level of response necessary;
- can help or suppress immune responses as necessary.

Autoimmunity can occur if any one of these jobs is not properly carried out or if the levels of different T cells become unbalanced, for example:

- if a particular immune response is amplified too much or for too long by hyperactive T helper cells;
- if the T suppressor cells fail to adequately damp down a vigorous response allowing it to continue long after it is needed.

Autoimmunity can occur through other T cell defects and recently it has been suggested that in patients with systemic lupus erythematosus, lymphocytes carrying the CD8 marker (conventionally thought of as T suppressor cells) actually encourage the production of autoantibodies.

Of course, one of the most important factors in determining whether an autoimmune disease will result from poorly functioning T cells is the precise nature of the antigens the immune response is directed against. If the response is to antigens that do not bear the slightest resemblance to normal body tissues then it is unlikely that an autoimmune state will result, no matter how poorly regulated the B cells are. However, if there is even a slight similarity between the antigen in question and body tissues (molecular mimicry) and the T cells fail to carry out their duties, then there is a stronger possibility that an autoimmune disease will occur.

Friendly fire

Recent studies on the heat shock proteins are relevant in this debate. These proteins are obvious targets for 'friendly fire' as the immune system confuses the invading micro-organism (antigen) with the body's own heat shock proteins. While firing at anything resembling the antigen, the immune system attacks the heat shock proteins. Research has suggested that this kind of reaction to heat shock proteins might be part of the damage process in rheumatoid arthritis, diabetes, and even systemic lupus erythematosus. More recently, however, a note of caution has been struck and the role of heat shock proteins in autoimmunity is undergoing a reappraisal.

T cell imbalance

How do the T cell populations become imbalanced in the first place? The level of T cells in the body is influenced by many factors:

- hormones;
- ageing;
- the expression of certain structures on the cell surface, such as the class II major histocompatibility complex molecules;
- drugs.

These factors can, in turn, be influenced by other factors, such as dietary fat, and thus the complexity of the autoimmune mosaic increases!

How complicated is the problem?

To illustrate further the complexity of a single factor affecting the immune system, consider the effect of diet. To be more precise, consider dietary fat, as an account of other aspects such as protein, calories, vitamins, and minerals could fill this entire book!

Fats are incorporated and used (metabolized) by the body in many different ways. It is sufficient to say that, after passing through the gut, different fats and oils are broken down into a fatty acid called arachidonic acid. This material is used in several important biochemical processes to generate other substances that regulate the immune system called leucotrienes and prostaglandins.

There are many different types of leucotrienes and prostaglandins, all of which can influence the outcome of immune responses—they can either induce inflammation or control and reduce it. Which of these responses they bring about seems to depend upon the type of fat entering the body as part of the diet. Generally high levels of saturated and unsaturated fat (a typical 'high fat' diet) promote the formation of inflammatory products, whereas other types of fat, such as fish oil, lead to the production of substances with anti-inflammatory properties.

Emerging from this rather complex picture is the suggestion that autoimmune responses can be influenced by diet (see Figure 4.5). While it is wrong to create too many expectations for nutritional therapy, there is no doubt that the intake of dietary fat can have a profound effect on the development of autoimmune disease in experimental animals. For example, when a certain type of laboratory mouse, which is prone to a lupus-like disorder, is fed from an early age either a low fat or a fish oil diet, the disease appears more slowly and the animals have a longer lifespan than animals placed on high fat diets. The animals fed a high fat diet also showed signs of serious immunological disorder at an early age.

A question of balance: yin–yang

Eastern philosophy uses the concept of yin–yang to represent the harmonious coexistence of opposing forces. The forces can be any pair of opposites: good and evil, rich and poor, health and disease. The concept has been extended to traditional Oriental medicine and is evident in such practices as acupuncture, where there is great emphasis on treating a condition by restoring 'balance' to the body rather than by simply alleviating the symptoms of disease. Such an approach has some merit and consideration of an immunological yin–yang is intriguing and perhaps relevant to the discussion of our mosaic model of autoimmune disease.

Autoimmunity results from an imbalance of the immunological forces in the body. We will now use one specific disease—rheumatoid arthritis— both in the context of the 'big picture', as before, and also in the context of yin–yang, to illustrate how an individual may develop a given autoimmune disorder.

Rheumatoid arthritis as a 'model' autoimmune disease

Infection may be an important trigger of the disease process in rheumatoid arthritis. Of course, only a minority of people who become infected, or who suffer some kind of joint injury (or both), will develop rheumatoid arthritis. This is because the immune system is, in fact, quite difficult to unbalance (see Figure 4.6).

A possible scheme of events that may result in an individual developing rheumatoid arthritis is shown in Figure 4.7.

An environmental cause?
Rheumatoid arthritis seems to be (in Europe at least) a disease of relatively recent times, which supports the notion that an infectious agent (a microorganism), introduced into the population, is an important trigger. If an infectious agent is important, what are the likely candidates? Both viruses and bacteria have been considered.

Viruses?
The Epstein–Barr virus has been the most likely suspect as a cause of rheumatoid arthritis. However, as most people have been infected with

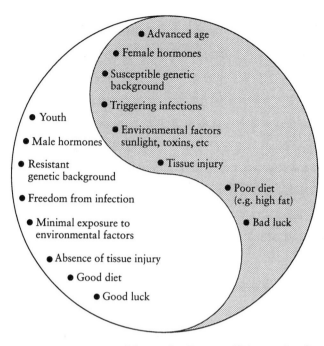

Figure 4.6 The yin–yang of factors leading to self-destructive disease.

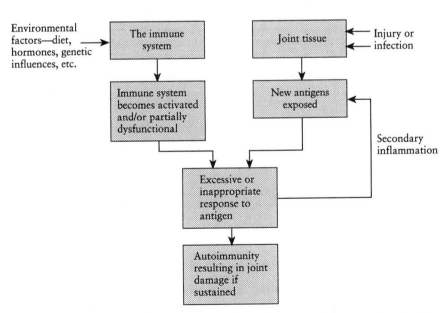

Figure 4.7 Scheme of events leading to the development of rheumatoid arthritis.

this virus by the time they reach adulthood, it is unclear why only a small proportion of individuals should develop the disease, and indeed some patients with rheumatoid arthritis have been shown not to have been infected with this virus.

Bacteria?

Many bacteria have been studied from the perspective of being triggers of autoimmune disease. In particular, the *Mycobacterium* family, which includes *Mycobacterium tuberculosis* (which causes tuberculosis), has been examined in great detail. However, it seems to be an unlikely factor in patients with rheumatoid arthritis as attempts to culture it from the joints of patients have generally been unsuccessful. However, there are many different forms of mycobacteria and a recent suggestion is that very slow growing forms may in fact be important triggers. There has also been a claim that another bacterium—*Proteus mirabilis*—might also be involved, although this claim remains controversial.

How do infectious agents act?

If infectious environmental agents are involved in diseases such as rheumatoid arthritis, it seems logical to assume that they would be involved in the triggering of the disease, rather than in its maintenance over many years. Molecular mimicry (Chapter 3, page 33) is a popular concept to explain the induction of autoimmune conditions. This phenomenon implies that an immune response to a foreign antigen (usually microbial), which happens by chance to resemble a self-antigen, induces an immune response against the self-antigen.

A genetic cause?

Genetic factors are important in rheumatoid arthritis—hospital-based studies have suggested a concordance rate for the disease in identical twins of approximately 30 per cent, compared with 5 per cent in non-identical twins. Although the figures in community-based studies are a little lower, the concept of a genetic factor in rheumatoid arthritis remains intact. However, these studies can also be interpreted as showing that several genes are important in predisposing an individual to rheumatoid arthritis.

Studies on Caucasian patients have found that approximately 70 per cent of patients had the human leucocyte antigen HLA DR4 marker on their lymphocytes. In contrast only 25 per cent of normal healthy subjects possessed this marker. Furthermore, patients with particularly severe rheumatoid arthritis were even more likely to be DR4-positive than those with less severe problems. The implication of this observation is that the presence of certain human leucocyte antigens on the lymphocytes may not only predispose an individual to developing rheumatoid arthritis but may also determine the type and severity of the disease.

The presence of human leucocyte antigen DR4 has been reported in other ethnic groups, including Japanese and Native North Americans, but it is not a universal marker. An Asian immigrant group in the UK has been found to have an increased frequency of human leucocyte antigen DR1 and, in at least one study of Greek patients, no human leukocyte antigen link could be found at all!

The human leucocyte antigens are involved in the trimolecular complex reaction, in which antigens that have been partially processed link together with the human leucocyte antigens and are recognized by receptors on T cells. An enormous amount of work has been done in the past few years to discover which amino acids make up the human leucocyte antigens that are involved in this process of antigen recognition. It now seems very likely that a small group of amino acids in an important position in the DR molecule predisposes an individual to rheumatoid arthritis. The precise relationship of these amino acids to the susceptibility for rheumatoid arthritis is not yet known. Detailed knowledge of the structure of this complex may enable the development of, for example, specific antibodies that block the function of the complex.

A local immune response?

Another suggestion, proposed in the mid-1980s, was that a local immune response to an environmental antigen could result in the release of cytokines (chemical messages) into the surrounding tissues (in the case of rheumatoid arthritis, the joints). This could in turn lead to the appearance, on the cell surface of certain cells, of human leucocyte antigens not usually present there. T cells might recognize these antigens and, if they also happen to bind to self-antigens, they could cause long-term chronic inflammation. However, if this mechanism is important in rheumatoid arthritis, then it is unclear which self-antigens are relevant.

Autoantibodies

Rheumatoid arthritis is not one single homogeneous disease and different forms clearly exist. Thus it is quite likely that several organisms can act as the trigger mechanism, possibly by activating the B cells and causing them to produce a 'burst' of many types of antibodies (including auto-antibodies). This autoimmune process would be maintained by the exposure of new autoantigens in the joint tissues. These may be unmasked by the initial wave of autoantibodies or by any trauma to the joint that may occur following an injury. Put in another way, minor tissue injury causes autoantigens not previously 'visible' to the immune system to be revealed. The immune system would recognize these antigens as foreign, and the sequence of activation and inflammation would take place. As a result, severe damage occurs within the joint tissues, often leaving the patient with the joint deformities typical of this disease.

The most widely recognized autoantibody in rheumatoid arthritis is rheumatoid factor. This immunoglobulin is a self-associating antibody, usually of the IgM class, which means that immunoglobulin M antibodies bind to part of the body's own immunoglobulin G (IgG) molecules. It is not known why rheumatoid factor is so often IgM, although IgG, IgA, and even IgE can also self-associate with IgG. High levels of IgM rheumatoid factor are relatively specific for patients with rheumatoid arthritis, although lower levels are found in a number of infectious and malignant diseases.

It has been shown that the lining of the joints in the hands, feet, wrists, and knees (where rheumatoid arthritis often occurs) contains cells that produce rheumatoid factor. Immune complexes of one antibody binding to another antibody are thus formed locally and may well be responsible, in part, for the chronic immunological damage that results in destruction of the joints.

Mechanisms of tissue damage in rheumatoid arthritis

The precise mechanisms by which various components of autoimmunity interact to cause the tissue damage seen in rheumatoid arthritis (and other autoimmune diseases) remain unclear. However, we are getting closer to being able to establish a reasonable reconstruction of events, especially those that occur once the disease has become established.

Most of the tissue damage in patients with rheumatoid arthritis is caused by lymphocytes or macrophages. Much work has been done to identify the chemical messengers that prompt these cells to pass into the joints. There are many different messengers, and certain components of the complement system are also important in 'summoning' the cells. This process is facilitated by the fact that lymphocytes detect or 'sniff out' the messenger molecules and follow their trail to the source in the tissue.

T cells

It seems very likely that T cells have an important role to play in the tissue damage in rheumatoid arthritis for the following reasons:

- Virtually no T cells are found in normal joints, whereas many are present in the joints of patients with rheumatoid arthritis.
- The T cells in the joints carry certain surface markers that suggest they are in an 'activated' state.
- Some of these T cells seem to have been selected because they bind to particular antigens.

Taken together, this evidence suggests that T cells are summoned to the joint and have a particular role to play.

B cells

The role of the B cells in the development of rheumatoid arthritis is based largely on their product, i.e. antibodies. As discussed, rheumatoid factors are known to be produced in the joint tissue and are likely to be involved in long-term damage. It is also evident that immunoglobulin G molecules in patients with rheumatoid arthritis lack a particular sugar—a defect also found in patients with tuberculosis (clearly an infectious disease) and Crohn's disease (an inflammatory disease of the bowel, which has long been suspected of having an infectious cause). These apparently distinct diseases may share common or related microbial trigger agents.

Macrophages and monocytes

Macrophages and monocytes are present in abundance in the joints of patients with rheumatoid arthritis. They appear in close association with another type of antigen presenting cell, known as dendritic cells, which are also over-represented in rheumatoid arthritis. Clearly the way in which these various cell types interact is critical to the development of inflammation in the joint and also to the development—it is not known why—of small lumps of tissue known as nodules, often found around the elbow joint in these patients.

Cytokines

Cytokines are important for many reasons, not least because they can control the growth of T cells and are also thought to play a role in the production of human leucocyte antigens.

The concentration of cytokines in the blood of patients with rheumatoid arthritis is often found to fluctuate, sometimes together with disease activity. However, levels of cytokines in the blood are not as important as the amounts produced locally in the joints which are clearly involved in maintaining inflammation there.

It appears that those cytokines produced predominantly by macrophages are particularly abundant and that those derived from T cells are less common.

Recent research has suggested that one particular cytokine — TNF alpha — may play a leading role in the inflammatory process. This observation is potentially important as antibodies to this cytokine might be of therapeutic benefit (see Chapter 6).

In a more general sense, the sooner we understand the precise interaction between inflammatory cells in the joints of patients with rheumatoid arthritis, the sooner we will be able to design more appropriate interventions to halt the progress of the disease.

The consequences of the inflammatory process

The presence of large numbers of inflammatory cells inside a joint has serious consequences. These cells release various enzymes that damage the cartilage inside the joint by breaking down its constituents. Cells that line the inside of many joints (synovial cells) are activated in response to this destruction and begin to multiply rapidly. They form a mass of tissue — the pannus — which actively invades and erodes both the cartilage and bone. The process is driven and sustained by the persisting influx of inflammatory cells, which release cytokines and the damaging enzymes. As the process gathers momentum the patient will notice swelling of the joints; this is often warm and very painful.

Summary

The events that lead to autoimmune conditions have not yet been defined precisely. From an immunological standpoint, it is likely that either:

- mechanisms that regulate the T cells are by-passed by newly exposed or altered self-antigens;
- autoantibody responses occur after infections.

In the second case, autoimmunity may result from the generalized activation of B cells or the production of antibodies that cross-react with self-antigens.

The events that trigger autoimmune disorders are also poorly under-stood; several species of microbe have been suggested as culprits but no single organism has emerged as a villain for any given disease. The overall consensus is that hormonal, microbial, genetic, and environmental factors need to act in concert for one of these disease to develop.

Apart from the events that may initiate one of these diseases, the factors that influence the type of disease and determine the organ-specificity of the autoimmune attack are also poorly understood. Why should one patient develop systemic lupus erythematosus, another rheumatoid arthritis, and another thyrotoxicosis? Why should one lupus patient develop severe renal disease and another cerebral involvement? The tissue damage that occurs in these diseases is usually attributed to the deposition of immune complexes but the factors that determine which organ will be attacked remain something of a mystery.

5

What can happen when the immune system tries to self destruct?

In this chapter each of the main autoimmune diseases will be described. Some, such as systemic lupus erythematosus and scleroderma, affect many different organs and systems (multisystemic) and can thus cause a wide variety of health problems. However, even diseases which are essentially confined to one organ or system may have widespread effects. A good example of this is diabetes mellitus in which the pancreas gland is the subject of the self-destructive attack. Since one of the principal functions of this gland is to secrete the hormone insulin which has many important roles throughout the body, any reduction in the rate of production leads to a wide variety of clinical features.

As well as a description of these diseases and the factors which conspire together to cause them, a brief outline of their treatment is provided. There are several exciting innovations in the treatment of autoimmune diseases that are currently being introduced for therapy.

What makes a disease autoimmune?

Thirty years ago, two American researchers (Milgrom and Witebsky) tried to answer this question by suggesting that various criteria should be met before any disease be referred to as autoimmune. In particular they proposed that a circulating antibody or cell-mediated immune response to a particular autoantigen should be identified for each disease. The auto-antigen itself should be identified. In an experimental animal model of the disease, it should be possible to transfer the condition by injecting the particular antibody or the self-reacting cells into another previously healthy animal. It should also be possible to produce the disease in an experimental animal by immunization with the self-antigen.

In truth, few diseases have met all of these criteria. For certain disorders described in this chapter, evidence of an autoimmune contribution remains controversial. Thus the evidence that scleroderma and inflammatory bowel disease are autoimmune in origin remains largely circumstantial. In some cases, such as ankylosing spondylitis, referred to earlier in the book, even the circumstantial evidence is weak and neither antibody- or cell-mediated responses have been identified. The linkage to autoimmunity thus remains tenuous.

Methods of classification

As indicated above, autoimmune diseases may be classified as either multi-systemic or mainly affecting one organ or system. Another way of trying to distinguish these disorders is by establishing whether they are caused principally by antibodies acting on their own, or as part of an immune complex with an antigen, and/or whether they are caused by cells. As each of the autoimmune diseases is discussed in turn, the category into which they fit most conveniently will be indicated.

Multisystem diseases

Systemic lupus erythematosus (SLE)

Systemic lupus erythematosus is perhaps the classic autoimmune disease, principally affecting women during the childbearing years, and most commonly giving rise to a skin rash, joint pain, and a profound sense of fatigue. The inflammation associated with lupus may also affect the heart, lungs, kidneys, and central nervous system. Although the mortality associated with lupus has greatly improved in the last 20 years, it remains a very troublesome condition for many patients, who often require treatment for months or years with major immunosuppressive drugs.

A short history

The name 'lupus' derives from the Latin meaning 'wolf' and refers to erythematous (red) ulcerations on the face. Systemic lupus erythematosus, while not acquiring its present name until the middle of the nineteenth century, was probably described by Hippocrates (460–370 BC). Lupus, while not as well known as, say, diabetes or rheumatoid arthritis, is perhaps the 'classic' autoimmune disease. Patients who suffer from it have abnormalities in virtually every compartment of their immune systems. However, the term lupus has been used to describe major skin conditions for at least seven centuries. Scholars such as Rogerius (c.1230), Paracelsus (1493–1541), Manardi (c.1500), and Sennert (1611) are all credited with mentioning lupus in their writings. Both Ferdinand von Hebra (1818–1880) and his son-in-law Moritz Kaposi (1872–1902) believed the 'herpes esthiomenos' of Hippocrates and the 'herpes ulcerosus' of Amatus Lusitanus (1510–65) to be synonyms for lupus.

The potentially serious nature of lupus has also been long recognized. Thus in 1813 Bateman commented that: 'Of this disease [lupus] I shall not treat at any length; for I can mention no medicine, which has been of any essential service in the cure of it ...'. He also described the facial distribution of the ulcerations. Laurent Biett (1781–1877) is credited by his pupils Pierre Cazenave (1795–1840) and Henri E. Schedel (1828, Paris), as describing the skin lesions of lupus with the term 'Erythema centrifugum' in 1828. By 1851, the term had become 'lupus arythemateux' (the latinized version being lupus erythematosus) and Cazenave described three principal varieties: '(1) Lupus which destroys the surface, (2) lupus which destroys in depth, and (3) lupus without ulcers but accompanied by hypertrophy of the involved parts.'

Von Hebra was possibly the first to liken the lupus rash to a butterfly. Although this skin problem was the first feature of lupus to be recorded, over the last 100 years the ability of the disease to mimic a wide variety of other conditions has been recognized. Thus Moritz Kaposi was the first to call attention to the seriousness of the condition and to recognize the systemic nature of lupus erythematosus. He understood that features such as fever, adenopathy (swelling of the lymph glands), and arthritis could be connected with the disease. Kaposi acknowledged that pleurisy, pneumonia, and disturbances of the central nervous system could also occur.

Between 1895 and 1903 William Osler, a physician born in Canada, published three papers expanding the concept that systemic lupus erythematosus was a systemic disease with complications. It is thought that the two young women described by Osler and who died of renal failure within 10 months of the appearance of a facial erythema, very probably had systemic lupus erythematosus. Osler published detailed descriptions of the women:

> ... arthritis, occasionally and a variable number of visceral [body] manifestations, of which the most important are gastrointestinal crises, endocarditis [inflammation of the inner layer of the heart], pericarditis [inflammation of the covering layer of the heart], acute nephritis [kidney inflammation] and haemorrhage from the mucosal surface. Recurrence is a special feature of the disease and attacks may come on month after month or even throughout a long period of years.

Features

The most common features of lupus are:

- skin rashes, which usually occur where the skin is exposed to light. These vary enormously, ranging from a minor red discoloration to enormous blisters;

- joint problems, which are generally pain and slight swelling, although major deformity can occur as a result of inflammation around the tendons;
- profound fatigue.

Other features include:

- involvement of the heart and lungs, usually due to a build-up of fluid in the tissues that support these organs. This can give rise to shortness of breath or pain when inhaling;
- central nervous system involvement, which is much more varied and difficult to describe. An enormous variety of symptoms, ranging from migraine to major epileptic fits, can develop. Major psychotic episodes can occur, as well as inflammation of the nerves which supply the face and limbs. The latter problem may cause loss of muscle power and normal sensation.

Lupus may also be responsible for the destruction of the body's own red and white blood cells and platelets. This can have a catastrophic effect, making the body more prone to infection, serious anaemia, and major bruising.

The lethargy experienced by lupus patients is often profound and disabling, patients frequently find it difficult to describe, as a result of which it is often disregarded by their family doctors. It is also common to find swelling of the lymph glands around the neck and in the armpits. Sometimes these have to be biopsied to make sure that no cancer has developed.

Autoimmune features

Many blood test abnormalities are also detectable in lupus patients, who often have antibodies that bind to many different components of the body. The best known of these autoantibodies are those that bind to DNA. It is generally believed that immune complexes consisting of DNA and anti-DNA antibodies are formed in the circulation of lupus patients and are deposited in the tissues. This deposition starts a chain of inflammatory events that results in kidney damage. There is also some evidence that anti-DNA antibodies may bind directly to the kidney tissue with similar consequences. A system of enzymes in the blood—the complement system (see Chapter 2)—which is usually activated to help protect the body against bacterial infection, often works overtime in patients with lupus, leading to exhaustion of some of its components. Repeated measurement of DNA antibodies and complement factors gives a guide to the patient's degree of active disease. It should be stressed, however, that it can sometimes be difficult to distinguish between the damage done by the disease in the past and the symptoms of active disease in the present. By analogy, a photograph of a village destroyed during a battle will not necessarily reveal if the battle which caused it to be destroyed is still raging.

Kidney disease
A major determinant of how lupus patients will fare is their degree of kidney disease. It is probably true to say that at least half of the patients with systemic lupus erythematosus have some degree of kidney involvement, but only about 10 per cent have severe disabling kidney disease. It is this group of patients which is most likely to do badly. The ten-year survival figure for lupus is around 85 per cent, but in the presence of severe kidney disease, this falls to around 70 per cent.

Prevalence
Systemic lupus erythematosus is largely confined to women during their child-bearing years. As discussed in Chapter 1, lupus is more common in black women (in the United States and the West Indies) than in Caucasian women (see Chapter 1, page 8).

A genetic cause?
The importance of the genetic component in lupus is strongly suggested by studies of similar and dissimilar twins. If one of a pair of identical twins has developed lupus, there is up to a 70 per cent chance that the other twin will also develop the disease; if the twins are dissimilar, the chance is around 10 per cent. While emphasizing the importance of the genetic component, this observation suggests that environmental factors must also be important. It has also been observed that between 2 and 4 per cent of the family members of lupus patients will develop the disease. This statistic is significantly higher than that among the normal population.

A hormonal cause?
The importance of hormones in the development of lupus is also critical. In most reports, women with lupus outnumber men by approximately 10 to 1, which strongly suggests a hormonal component as an important factor.

Other causes
Ultraviolet light may trigger a flare-up of the disease and there are certain drugs (notably some used in the treatment of high blood pressure) which

can bring on a milder variant of this disease. Common viral infections may also be responsible for the onset or flare up of lupus.

Treatment

There is no cure for systemic lupus erythematosus but in the majority of patients the symptoms can be controlled successfully. Its milder symptoms can be helped by non-steroidal or antimalarial drugs. The use of anti-malarials was the result of a chance observation and why these drugs should help to combat the lethargy, joint pain, and skin rashes in many lupus patients remains uncertain.

Steroids

Steroids are invariably required when patients develop serious involvement of their heart and lungs. The use of these drugs is not an easy option, as the side-effects of over treatment are serious and include:

- thinning of the bones (osteoporosis);
- diabetes mellitus;
- high blood pressure;
- an increased risk of infection.

Nevertheless, despite these potential side-effects (described in more detail in Chapter 6), steroids may be life-saving and certainly help to control most manifestations of the disease. Their mechanism of action is discussed in Chapter 6.

Combination drug therapy

Unfortunately, steroids on their own may be insufficient and many patients will require a combination of steroids and other drugs to suppress their overactive immune system. These drugs (notably azathioprine and cyclo-phosphamide; see Chapter 6) may be given by mouth or, in the case of cyclophosphamide, by slow intravenous injection. This 'infusion' method is popular in the USA, but is not used to the same extent in the UK. It too may have major side-effects, as described in Chapter 6.

Plasma exchange

Plasma exchange (plasmapheresis; see Chapter 6 for details) is sometimes beneficial. Blood is removed from a patient's vein and passed through a machine that separates the components of the blood. The plasma is removed because it contains the antibodies which are thought to be harmful in this condition. By removing these antibodies, especially if the patient is also on immunosuppressive drugs, it is hoped that the self-destructive forces will not be able to successfully regroup and mount another attack. The blood cells are returned to the patient's bloodstream together with fresh plasma from a healthy volunteer. However, this is a very expensive procedure and many patients experience a 'rebound' of their symptoms after a few weeks.

Rheumatoid arthritis

Although many organs and systems can be affected by rheumatoid arthritis, it causes principally inflammation of the small joints of the hands and feet, often in a symmetrical fashion, giving rise to swelling and pain. The condition mainly affects women, usually starting between the ages of 30 and 55, and often lasts for several decades.

History

There is some disagreement about how long rheumatoid arthritis has affected the human population. Examination of Saxon skeletons and the bony remains of ancient Egyptians has shown clear evidence of osteo-arthritis (the 'wear and tear' arthritis associated with old age) and spondy-litis (a condition affecting the lower back, which starts as inflammation of the supporting ligaments and leads to severe stiffness of the spine), but there is very little archaeological evidence of rheumatoid arthritis. Some authorities believe that rheumatoid arthritis was brought back from the New World by the early explorers. Support for this hypothesis comes from Monte Alban in Mexico, an ancient site originally occupied by Zapotec Indians. In the ruins of the 2000-year-old Temple of the Dancers are stone slabs depicting the ill and the deformed, including figures with swollen hands and feet.

Although Botticelli is thought to have depicted rheumatoid arthritis-like deformities in some of the subjects of his paintings in the fifteenth century (see Figures 5.1 and 5.2), the first detailed case report of the disease was by a French medical student—Augustin Jacob Landré-Beauvais—who, in 1827, described a frail 35-year-old woman with multiple joint swelling that settled gradually, leaving her with deformed wrists and hands, but which recurred later.

The question of the origin of rheumatoid arthritis is not yet resolved, but it does appear that, in Europe at least, it is a disorder of relatively modern times. This is a striking observation given its relative frequency (almost 1 per cent of the Caucasian population, although more recent

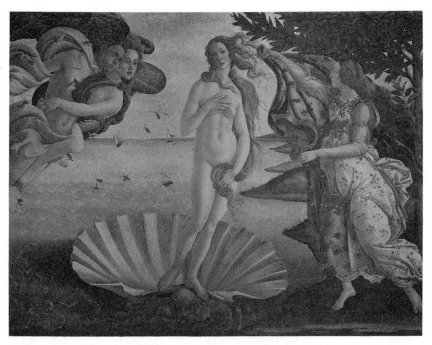

Figure 5.1 *The Birth of Venus*: Sandro Botticelli: (Uffizi Gallery, Florence). Venus' right-hand fingers appear swollen.

studies suggest that it is becoming less common) and has in turn led to reflections upon a possible microbial contribution to its cause.

Rheumatoid arthritis is an inflammatory condition that usually affects the synovial joints—hands, wrists, elbows, shoulders, knees, hips, ankles, and small foot joints. These joints are lined with a special membrane (the synovial membrane), which secretes a type of 'oil' to keep them lubricated. The process by which the joints end up being badly damaged is illustrated in Chapter 4. An inflammatory mass of tissue (a pannus) forms inside the joints and erodes the adjacent bone and cartilage.

The severity of the disease

There are several types of rheumatoid arthritis, ranging from a relatively mild self-limiting disease, to a severe deforming arthritis for which all forms of treatment appear to be ineffectual. The majority of patients have a slow, remitting and relapsing, or chronic persistent condition, in which there is destruction of the joints with erosion of the bone beneath. This process leads to the deformities in the small joints of the hands and feet, as well as some of the bigger joints.

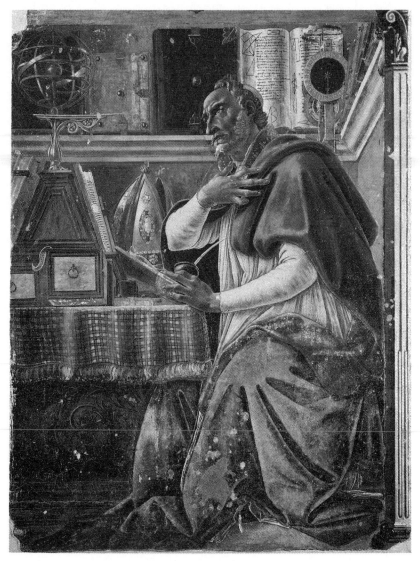

Figure 5.2 *St Agostino*: Sandro Botticelli (Chiesa di Oganissanti, Florence). Here the joints on both the subject's hands appear swollen.

Features

Among the general features and complications of rheumatoid arthritis are:

- weight loss;
- thinning of the skin with increased risk of ulceration;
- dryness of the eyes or mouth;

- inflammation of the peripheral nerves, which may produce numbness in the hands and feet.

Effects on the spinal cord

Of particular importance is the joint in the spine linking the first and second neck vertebrae. The pannus that forms in the joints here may put pressure on the spinal cord. This can have devastating consequences, including complete loss of the use of the arms and legs. Fortunately, this complication is relatively unusual, and modern surgery can usually prevent the problem before it is too late.

Blood abnormalities

The major abnormality found in the blood of patients with rheumatoid arthritis is the presence of rheumatoid factor (see page 72)—an antibody that binds to part of another human immunoglobulin (IgG). As discussed in detail in Chapter 4, there is evidence of both immune complex and cellular abnormalities in the development of rheumatoid arthritis. Rheumatoid factors can also be produced in a whole host of other infectious and autoimmune diseases. Its precise function in patients with infectious disease remains unknown, as is its significance in the development of rheumatoid arthritis.

Treatment

There is no simple and effective treatment for rheumatoid arthritis. In the past, some of the drugs used were described as 'disease-modifying', although it is not certain how drugs like gold, penicillamine, chloroquine, or the more recently introduced sulphasalazine can 'modify' the disease. However, they may be able to halt its advance for a while and provide some relief from the symptoms of pain and swelling.

All of these drugs have potential side-effects; gold and penicillamine which can give rise to kidney damage, skin rashes, and bone marrow suppression (preventing the normal production of cells in the blood) are probably the most toxic.

The immunosuppressive drug methotrexate is widely used in the USA for the treatment of the more severe forms of rheumatoid arthritis. It appears to be successful in halting the progression of disease in many patients although its side-effects (liver damage, bone marrow suppression, and rashes) may limit its use. Azathioprine (another immunosuppressive drug) is also prescribed for many patients but other types of treatment such as total lymph node irradiation and plasma exchange (see Chapter 6, page 115 for details) have largely been abandoned.

Sjögren's syndrome

This condition causes profound dryness of the eyes or mouth, is much more common in women than men, and is usually treated symptomatically. Many patients with Sjögren's syndrome also have arthritis and a variety of autoantibodies in their blood.

Henrik Sjögren was the first person to describe the combination of dryness of the eyes and mouth in patients with rheumatoid arthritis. He described a number of such cases in his research thesis, which was published in German in 1933. It was not widely read and, unfortunately, when it was translated into English in 1943 other more major world events ensured that it received little attention. Nevertheless, during the 1950s and 1960s, Sjögren's descriptions were gradually accepted.

There are different types of Sjögren's syndrome. Those patients with the symptoms of dryness who also have another autoimmune disease (such as rheumatoid arthritis or lupus) are said to have secondary Sjögren's. However, the same symptoms may occur on their own, which is known as primary Sjögren's syndrome. The vagina may also be extremely dry. The disease usually begins before menopause but some symptoms of the menopause itself may be difficult to distinguish from Sjögren's syndrome. The disorder is further complicated by frequent joint pains, although unlike rheumatoid arthritis these are not associated with any major joint deformity. The symptoms of primary Sjögren's syndrome are accompanied by a variety of blood test abnormalities. For example, half of these patients have rheumatoid factors and nearly 90 per cent have antinuclear antibodies. Patients with Sjögren's syndrome often have high levels of circulating immune complexes and among the antinuclear antibodies found those binding to combinations of RNA and protein known as Ro and La (the letters come from the first letters of the surnames of the patients in whom the antibodies were first found) are particularly prominent. However, the major problem with Sjögren's patients is that the salivary glands (in the mouth), the lacrimal glands (in the eyes), and glands elsewhere in the body that keep various body surfaces damp, are infiltrated by self-reacting cells, mostly lymphocytes and macrophages. It is the invasion by these cells that results in the destruction of those parts of the glands that secrete fluid and thus cause the symptoms of dryness. Rheumatoid factors are also produced within the glands of patients with Sjögren's syndrome and are thus part of the ongoing inflammatory process.

Abnormalities of the nervous system occur but, although unpleasant, these are relatively mild, including some loss of feeling in the hands and feet. Tingling in the thumb and first two fingers may occur and is due to increased pressure on the nerve that passes over the wrist joint to supply these fingers.

Patients with Sjögren's syndrome have an increased risk of a malignant change in their lymphocytes. This may give rise to a type of cancer known as lymphoma, which requires major cytotoxic therapy (see page 113).

For most patients, Sjögren's syndrome is a 'nuisance' disease, for which symptomatic treatment—eye drops, mouth washes, and vaginal lubricants —is all that is needed. However, corticosteroid treatment is sometimes required.

Scleroderma

The term 'scleroderma' comes from the Latin meaning 'hard skin'; it is a particularly unpleasant but uncommon disease. It is largely confined to women and usually starts in the skin of the fingers. The skin becomes hardened, thickened, and has poor circulation so that in cold weather the hands will undergo a striking white, blue, then red colour change. The poor circulation component is known as Raynaud's syndrome, but this is not confined to scleroderma and usually occurs on its own. The changes in the skin may move rapidly up the arms and may involve great swathes across the chest wall; the legs may also be involved. The joints become stiff and there may be an accompanying inflammation within the muscles. In severe cases it may be difficult to open the mouth to eat solid food.

These features alone would be bad enough but scleroderma may also affect some of the internal organs, in particular the intestinal tract. This complication often manifests as a hiatus hernia, with acid passing from the stomach back up into the oesophagus. The large bowel may also be affected so that faeces cannot be moved. Rarely, this is so severe that patients may open their bowels just once or twice a month! The result is extremely painful and may require surgery to remove the affected bowel.

Like systemic lupus, scleroderma may affect the heart, lungs, and kidneys. Kidney disease is particularly serious and may be life threatening.

While scleroderma is not a classic autoimmune disease, abnormal immune function is an integral part of its pathology. Disease-specific autoantibodies of several types have been identified in patients with scleroderma but their role in the development of the disease is uncertain. In early stages of the disease, when it involves the skin or internal organs, cells migrate from the blood vessels and form large collections of lymphocytes, plasma cells, and macrophages in the affected tissues. Three different types of auto-antibodies are virtually confined to these patients and, some studies have also reported abnormal T lymphocyte cell function in these patients.

Treatment

There is no cure and although a number of drugs such as steroids, D-penicillamine, or colchicine are prescribed, they are of limited benefit. Indeed, there is a medical saying that no new drug can be said to be entirely useless until it has been tried in the treatment of scleroderma! However, many patients have a limited form of the disease and it is now recognized that scleroderma may very occasionally go into a spontaneous remission. In addition, many aspects of the disease can be helped, thus the severe Raynaud's phenomenon that troubles many patients can be eased greatly by taking care to avoid exposure to the cold unless wearing gloves. Electrically heated gloves and other local aids are available. Drugs which dilate the blood vessels may be given successfully by mouth or, in severe cases, by intravenous infusion.

Diseases confined to one organ or system

Insulin-dependent diabetes mellitus (type I)

Type I insulin-dependent diabetes mellitus usually begins between the ages of 10 and 20 and follows an autoimmune attack upon cells in the pancreas gland. The immediate clinical features are increased thirst and the passing of large amounts of water with a high sugar content. In later years damage to the kidneys, blood vessels throughout the body, and central nervous system are well recognized complications which may be difficult to treat.

Another type of diabetes mellitus (type II) occurs later in life and is often associated with being overweight. It does not usually require insulin treatment and is not thought to be autoimmune in origin.

History

The term 'diabetes' comes from the Greek, meaning 'to run through a syphon', and was first used by Aretaeus of Cappadocia (AD 81–138), who noted the large amount of urine (polyuria) associated with this disease. However, polyuria (excessive amounts of urine) had been recognized as a feature of diabetes much earlier. A papyrus dating from about 1550 BC, found in a grave in Thebes by the Egyptologist George Ebers, contains a description of several diseases including a polyuric state resembling diabetes. It also seems likely that Japanese and Chinese physicians of the second and third centuries were well aware of both the polyuria and of the sweet taste of the urine in patients with the disease. Similarly, old Sanskrit texts from India written during the fifth and sixth centuries BC refer to 'urine of honey'. The widespread distribution of this disease is further indicated by the descriptions of several Arab physicians, who recorded the sweetness of urine, abnormal appetite, propensity for gangrene, and loss of sexual function that are well known symptoms of diabetes.

Paradoxically, there are few European references to diabetes during the Middle Ages, although the impressively named German physician Aureolus Theophrastus Bombastus von Hochenheim (1493–1541) described how he evaporated the urine of a diabetic patient and obtained a white powdery residue. Unfortunately, Dr von Hochenheim's astute observation was marred by the fact that he mistook the isolated substance for salt instead of sugar! Matthew Dobson, a physician in Liverpool (1735–84), was the first to prove that the urine of diabetic patients really did contain sugar and to suggest that it probably came originally from the serum rather than being formed in the kidneys.

It was an English physician, William Colum (1710–90) who added the term 'mellitus' to diabetes, in order to distinguish it from another form known as 'diabetes insipidus', which is due to damage of the pituitary gland in the brain.

It was only more recently that therapeutic measures were tried with any degree of success. Apollinaire Bouchardat (1806–86) noted that the famine caused by the siege of Paris during the Franco-Prussian war of 1870 was associated with an improvement in the condition of many of his diabetic patients (see page 47). However, it was not until the end of the nineteenth century that damage to the pancreas was linked to diabetes mellitus. Eventually experiments in dogs showed that the complete removal of the pancreas led to diabetes. The successful isolation of the blood sugar lowering hormone (insulin) derived from a component of the pancreas, known as the islets of Langerhans, which contain the beta islet cells, by Banting and Best in 1921 was the key observation which has led to the alleviation of many of the terrible effects of diabetes.

The pancreas (the word is derived from the Greek meaning 'sweet bread') is a small, elongated gland situated beneath the stomach. It secretes pancreatic juice, which helps to digest food, into the intestine. It also produces the hormone insulin, which is vital in the control of carbohydrate metabolism and, in particular, makes sure that the level of glucose in the blood remains relatively constant. Without sufficient insulin the level of glucose in the blood rises and, if not corrected in time, this may result in greatly increased thirst, excessive production of urine, and eventually to coma. Diabetes mellitus is now known to be the result of damage to small cells, known as beta islet cells, that are normally found in clusters within the pancreas.

Cause

The cause of insulin-dependent diabetes is uncertain, but it seems likely that, in a susceptible individual, infection of the insulin-producing pancreas cells by a virus can lead to some form of self-perpetuating auto-immune damage.

There is compelling evidence of genetic predisposition to diabetes mellitus. Thus 90 to 95 per cent of Caucasians with the disease have the human leucocyte antigen DR3, or DR4, or both (compared with approximately 50 per cent of the general population). If one of a pair of identical twins develops lupus there is a 40 to 50 per cent chance that the other twin will get the disease. In contrast if the twins are not identical the risk is only 5 to 10 per cent. This too suggests that genetic factors are important in the development of the disease but does imply that other factors are essential.

Antibodies that can bind to the islet cells in the pancreas are strongly associated with diabetes. These antibodies may develop months or even years before the clinical symptoms of diabetes develop. By the time of diagnosis these antibodies are present in up to 90 per cent of diabetics. However, whether they are really an essential part of the process that ends up destroying the insulin-producing cells is uncertain; most authorities believe that cell-mediated mechanisms are probably more important. The precise sequence of events and knowledge of which particular cells are involved in the long-term damage to the pancreas remain to be determined.

Treatment

The traditional method of treatment is to inject insulin two or three times a day. This is not ideal because, under normal circumstances, the amount of insulin released by the pancreas depends upon the level of glucose in the blood and is carefully monitored by the healthy functioning gland.

For many years the insulin that was used to treat diabetics was derived from animal sources, notably the cow and the pig. In the hopes of providing a more natural product, genetically engineered human insulin was introduced a few years ago. Unexpectedly, this has proved to be of dubious benefit in some patients, who experience dramatic falls in blood sugar levels, leading to light-headedness or even collapse. For this reason, newer techniques of infusing insulin into the body with more frequent checks of the blood glucose are being introduced. They hold the key to a healthier future for diabetics.

Autoimmune thyroid disease

There are two forms of self-destructive thyroid disease, one of which— Graves' disease—is associated with overproduction of the thyroid hormone (thyroxine) while the other—Hashimoto's disease—is associated with a reduction in levels of this hormone.

History

The history of autoimmune thyroid disease predates the discovery that the condition is a result of a self-destructive process. Again, a key observation linking the clinical features of a disease with the removal of a gland led to rapid advances. Thus in 1883 Reverdin and Cochin showed that the removal of the thyroid gland was associated with the features that are generally referred to as myxoedema (underactive thyroid). In 1891 it was reported, by Murray, that injection of a thyroid extract could relieve the symptoms of low thyroid hormone production. Within two years, Horwitz used lightly cooked sheep thyroid glands to successfully treat myxoedema.

The thyroid gland, situated at the base of the neck, produces a hormone called thyroxine, whose role is most easily understood as the facilitator for a wide range of metabolic processes in most tissues. It is thus a sort of 'oil in the machinery' essential for the normal functioning of muscles, bone growth, and mental function, among other things. The thyroid is the victim of two forms of autoimmune attack:

- Hashimoto's thyroiditis;
- Graves' disease.

Hashimoto's thyroiditis

In Hashimoto's thyroiditis, there is chronic inflammation of the thyroid gland, associated with antibodies to several thyroid components, with underproduction of thyroxine. This condition is also called myxoedema. Autoantibodies against two major components of the thyroid gland (thyroglobulin and thyroid microsomes) are clinically the most important for diagnosis. Although levels of these antibodies in the blood correlate well with disease activity they do not transfer the disease when injected into healthy animals. One theory of how Hashimoto's thyroiditis develops suggests that the antibodies alone or as part of an immune complex bind to cells within the thyroid and that these cells are later destroyed by 'killer' lymphocyte cells (which recognize the Fc portion (see page 22) of the bound antibodies).

Features
The classic features are severe lethargy, dry skin and hair, and damage to the nerves in the limbs. These patients often require long-term thyroid hormone replacement. The ratio of women to men is approximately 5 to 1; the condition usually occurs in middle life and is treated by taking thyroxine tablets.

Graves' disease
Graves' disease is associated with overactivity of the thyroid gland. Patients have antibodies that bind to and stimulate hormone receptors on the surface of the thyroid gland; this increases the production of thyroxine by the gland. These receptors are usually occupied by thyroid-stimulating hormone, which is produced by the pituitary gland and is the natural regulator of thyroid hormone levels. By occupying the thyroid-stimulating hormone receptors in the thyroid gland, the autoantibodies trick the thyroid into thinking it is receiving a message from the pituitary gland to increase its production of thyroxine. As a result the thyroid gland, and consequently the patient, become hyperactive.

Features
Patients with Graves' disease often have protruding eyeballs, giving the eyes a striking, staring look. These patients, frequently women in their forties (the female to male ratio is 7 to 1) usually complain of weight loss, anxiety, tremor of the hands, and can have a fast pulse and express an extreme dislike for hot weather.

Treatment
The condition can be treated successfully by controlling the overactive thyroid with antithyroid drugs, radioactive iodine, or surgery; combinations of these treatments have proved very successful.

Multiple sclerosis
This is an inflammatory disease of the white matter of the central nervous system that results in progressive neurological defects, including impaired vision, unsteadiness of the limbs and loss of feeling of different parts of the skin. It remains a very difficult condition to treat successfully.

This is the most common crippling disease of the nervous system to affect young adults, especially in Caucasian populations. The condition is often characterized by relapses and remissions; each relapse tends to increase the amount of permanent damage done to the nervous system.

The disease takes many, often bizarre forms. In a matter of hours, or days, patients may lose vision or the use of arms or legs, develop a tremor or stiffness in the limbs, with marked unsteadiness. The symptoms will often resolve over a period of weeks or months, only to be followed by further attacks as time goes by. The outcome for individual patients is unpredictable. Some become permanently disabled, a few are confined to a wheelchair, while others have occasional attacks and are able to live normal lives most of the time.

Most nerves are coated by a protein called myelin, which is responsible for the rapid progress of nervous impulses around the body. In multiple sclerosis the nerves lose their myelin coating (a process known as de-myelination) (Figure 5.3)—this occurs in scattered patches throughout the nervous system. These scattered patches of demyelination contain inflammatory cells, notably T cells and macrophages. The inflammation caused by these cells destroys the myelin and interferes with the normal passage of nerve impulses by reducing the effectiveness of nerve transmission. It is the cause of the many symptoms of this disease—the patient may have muscle weakness, progressive paralysis, or a loss of normal sensation.

Multiple sclerosis is more common among young females and the

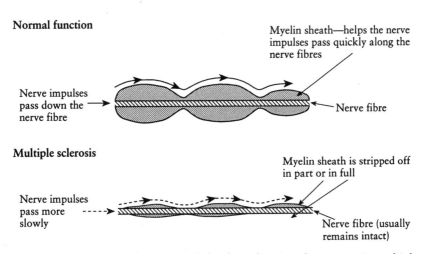

Figure 5.3 Normal myelination and the demyelination that occurs in multiple sclerosis.

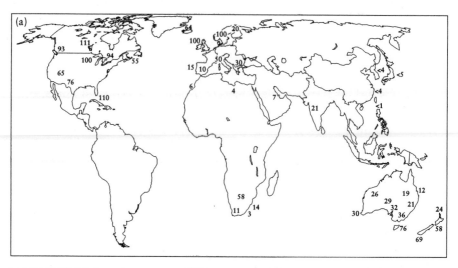

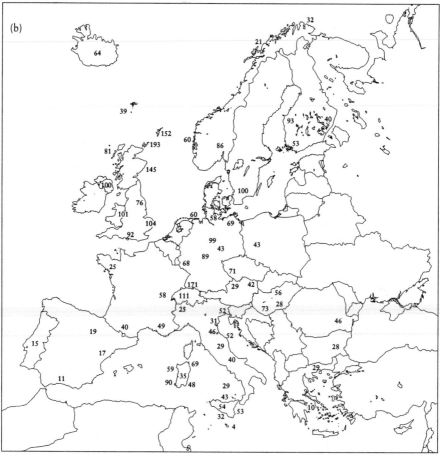

Figure 5.4 Estimates for the prevalence (per 10^5) of multiple sclerosis (a) throughout the world and (b) in Europe (1975–1989). The figures are taken from published sources and have been derived using methods that are not necessarily comparable (copyright *Journal of the Royal College of Physicians of London*).

prevalence displays a curious pattern (Figure 5.4). It is common in northern Europe, North America, and Australia, but rare in the Far East, Asia, India and Pakistan, Africa, and South America. Studies of the movements of migrating northern Europeans have suggested that there are important genetic and environmental influences—if, after the age of 15, individuals move from a high risk to a low risk area they retain an increased chance of developing the disease.

Magnetic resonance imaging (an image produced by placing part of the body inside a large magnet) has proved a very useful test for demonstrating the scattered areas (plaques) of demyelination in the nervous system. Other useful tests for helping to make the diagnosis include measuring the immunoglobulin level in the fluid that surrounds the brain and spinal cord (if it is raised this suggests that autoantibodies are being over produced locally); assessing the cerebrospinal fluid (obtained by a lumbar puncture), and performing electrical stimulation tests of the eyes and ears (which are impaired if there is a loss of myelin around the nerve sheaths).

Treatment

Many types of treatment have been prescribed for multiple sclerosis, although none is of much help. Corticosteroids have been shown to shorten the duration of an acute attack and intensive immunosuppressive therapy with drugs like azathioprine, cyclophosphamide, and antilymphocyte globulin has been tried. Plasma exchange (plasmapheresis) has also been attempted, but to date the results are generally disappointing. Trials of combined immunosuppressive therapies are being explored. Adequate rest and the avoidance of stress are usually advised to help prevent a relapse.

Myasthenia gravis

As the name (Latin for 'serious muscle weakness') implies, this is a chronic, progressive muscular weakness; it may occur at any time between infancy and old age and may affect any ethnic group. It usually begins in the face and throat but is not often associated with muscle wasting. It was first described clinically by the physiologist Thomas Willis.

Myasthenia gravis is closely related to thyrotoxicosis and the two diseases occur together more frequently than can be expected by chance. Furthermore, this condition is associated on occasion with diabetes mellitus, rheumatoid arthritis and systemic lupus erythematosus. These simple observations prompted the Scottish physician, John Simpson, to speculate, in 1960, that myasthenia gravis might be an autoimmune disease. It is now arguably the best understood of all human autoimmune diseases and has served as a model to help understand the mechanisms which induce other such disorders.

In this condition, antibodies are formed to a receptor for the chemical transmitter acetylcholine, which passes electrical impulses from the nerves to the muscles. The antireceptor antibodies bind to the receptors and so reduce the number of receptors available for acetylcholine. This makes it harder for nerve impulses to stimulate the muscles into action. The failure of transmission of the nerve impulse at many junctions means that the power of the whole muscle is reduced, thus causing the weakness which is the main clinical feature of the disease. Much of the research done in this field has used receptors obtained from the electric eel. Indeed a major advance in our understanding of myasthenia was made in 1973 when Patrick and Lindstrom immunized rabbits with electric eel acetylcholine receptors. The rabbits developed muscular weakness similar to that seen in humans with myasthenia gravis; the weakness was shown to be due to antibodies directed against the receptor. Later studies showed that antibodies from an affected animal would induce the disease, usually within 48 hours after injection into a healthy animal. Thus myasthenia gravis meets all of the criteria for an autoimmune disease put forward by Milgrom and Witebsky that were discussed at the start of the chapter (see page 76).

Patients with myasthenia gravis complain how easily their muscles seem to feel 'tired'. They find that they cannot contract their muscles for long periods. Thus the classic features are drooping of the eyelids, slowing of speech, and, more worryingly, breathing difficulties in severe cases. Myasthenia gravis affects 50–125 people per million of the population and about 25 000 cases are estimated to be present in the United States (about one-seventh the number with lupus erythematosus).

There are two types of myasthenia gravis (three if one counts a transient form occurring in the newborn children of mothers with the disease). The 'early onset' type is found mainly in females under the age of forty, whereas the 'late onset' variety is found equally distributed in men as women over this age. In the younger onset group there is a strong association with human leucocyte antigen A1, B8, and DR3; the same profile as for many lupus patients. In the older onset group there is a weaker link with B7 and DR2.

Abnormalities in the thymus gland are found in almost three-quarters of patients with myasthenia gravis. In 10 per cent of affected individuals a form of tumour—a thymoma—develops in the thymus gland. Removal of the thymus gland, especially in the early stages of the disease, can help to relieve or even cure the symptoms. It has been suggested that the initial abnormal immune response in myasthenia may be against acetylcholine receptors on epithelial cells in the thymus, and that there is some form of cross-reactivity (similarity in structure) between the acetylcholine receptors in the thymus and in the muscles.

Treatment

Many drugs are available to help stimulate the muscles. These drugs block the action of an enzyme, cholinesterase, that normally destroys acetylcholine. Thus they act to increase the amount of acetylcholine in the body. On occasion, steroids and azathioprine may be helpful. For very severe cases life support machines are required during acute attacks but the majority of cases can be well controlled and the disease is rarely life-threatening.

Myositis

Myositis is a rare disease causing weakness of the muscles, especially those moving the shoulders and hips. It affects approximately three times as many women as men and it is most commonly found between the ages of 40 and 60. A childhood form can occur, which is associated in particular with a skin rash on the eyelids and sometimes over the knuckles and forearms.

In myositis, there is inflammation and destruction of the skeletal muscles. Patients thus have difficulty standing, getting out of a chair, and raising their arms. Myositis can be life-threatening if the muscles involved in swallowing and breathing are affected.

As muscle destruction occurs, enzymes are released into the blood from the damaged tissue; levels may rise 10 to 50 times greater than normal. An example is the enzyme creatinine kinase which is of importance in normal muscle contraction. Certain characteristic autoantibodies to components of the cell nucleus are also present. These antibodies bind to other enzymes concerned with the normal formation of proteins. However, why these antibodies develop is at present unknown.

Treatment

Most patients can be treated successfully with steroids and other drugs that suppress the immune system, although perhaps 20 per cent do not respond. For this latter group of patients there is a very real danger of falling over, which can be very serious, causing broken bones and internal bleeding.

Pernicious anaemia

Pernicious anaemia is a relatively common condition, mostly affecting middle-aged women. These patients have antibodies to some of the cells of the stomach lining and to the binding sites concerned with the absorption of vitamin B12. As a consequence, the absorption of this important vitamin is impaired and a characteristic form of anaemia with enlarged red blood cells results. Patients with this disease become weak and may develop numbness or weakness of the hands and feet.

Treatment

Pernicious anaemia can be treated successfully by regular injections of vitamin B12.

Autoimmune haemolytic anaemia and thrombocytopenia

Destruction of the body's own red blood cells due to the formation of antibodies against them may occur in patients with systemic lupus erythematosus or on its own. Another type of blood cell, the platelets (which are normally involved in blood clotting), can also be the subject of an autoimmune attack. A low level of platelet cells is known as thrombocytopenia.

When acute and severe, haemolytic anaemia and thrombocytopenia are life threatening. Anaemia causes a feeling of exhaustion and a pale complexion, whereas low platelet numbers mean that the skin and, more worryingly, the internal organs bruise and bleed easily.

Treatment

Both conditions require treatment with steroids, often in high doses, and sometimes accompanied by other major immunosuppressive drugs.

Primary biliary cirrhosis/chronic active hepatitis

The liver may be the target of several forms of autoimmune attack. Two such examples are primary biliary cirrhosis and chronic active hepatitis. Primary biliary cirrhosis is the result of a chronic inflammatory process in the liver, causing destruction of its normal architecture and resulting in swelling of the gland and also some damage to the spleen.

Patients with either of these conditions often have jaundice, enlargement of the liver, and severe itching. Primary biliary cirrhosis is largely confined to middle-aged women and chronic active hepatitis to younger women. Both conditions have a chronic inflammatory process which gives rise to destructive changes within the liver. The diseases are distinguished by differences in their antibody profiles and in their response to steroids.

Treatment
Chronic active hepatitis usually responds to steroid treatment; primary biliary cirrhosis does not.

Pemphigus
Pemphigus and its less severe variant, pemphigoid, are the result of an autoimmune process affecting the skin and are characterized by large blisters that appear without warning. These diseases mostly occur in middle aged and elderly people. On occasion pemphigus occurs as part of the spectrum of other forms of autoimmune disease including lupus, rheumatoid arthritis, and myasthenia gravis.

Treatment
Pressure over the skin may induce a blister and the condition may be serious enough to require large doses of steroids. Other immunosuppressive drugs may be required, and sometimes plasma exchange is used as well. This condition carries a variable and uncertain prognosis.

Other autoimmune diseases

Goodpasture's syndrome
The kidney may be involved in an autoimmune attack as part of a multi-systemic disease such as systemic lupus erythematosus or may be the only organ involved in such an attack. In Goodpasture's syndrome, antibodies that bind to the lining cells in the kidney (and also the lung) are formed. These autoantibodies bind to structures in the lining or basement membrane parts of the kidneys and lungs. Thus immune complexes are formed in these organs, the complement system (see Chapter 3) is activated, and lymphocytes and macrophages are 'attracted' into the tissues, causing inflammation and damage. In a healthy person the kidney serves a crucial role by acting as a filter that removes waste products from the bloodstream.

In Goodpasture's syndrome, a rapidly progressive form of inflammation, known as glomerulonephritis, often develops. This results in the kidney becoming 'leaky' and allowing a variety of blood cells and proteins to escape into the urine. High blood pressure and the generally debilitated state associated with kidney failure may develop unless treatment is started promptly. Damage in the lung often leads to coughing up blood-stained sputum. Without treatment, Goodpasture's syndrome may lead to death within weeks or months, but it has been shown that plasma exchange may be life-saving in this condition.

Glomerulonephritis

The kidney is a target for two types of disease that follow from antibodies accumulating in an organ. Thus the autoantibodies may bind directly to target antigens in the kidney itself (Goodpasture's syndrome is a good example of this). Alternatively, antibodies, as part of an immune complex circulating in the blood, may become deposited or lodged in the kidney tissue. This may occur in patients with systemic lupus erythematosus (see page 77), in whom circulating immune complexes, consisting of DNA and anti-DNA antibodies, have been identified and are thought to be a major instigator of inflammation and damage in the kidneys. A wider variety of immune complex constituents has been identified in different conditions. For example, some patients with autoimmune thyroid disease develop kidney disease as a result of the deposition of immune complexes consisting of thyroglobulin and anti-thyroglobulin antibodies.

The chain of events that follows the deposition of antibody, by either method, varies somewhat according to the precise location of the deposits. Clinically, the result is usually some form of glomerulonephritis, literally inflammation of the kidney glomeruli, which are the filtering units through which the kidney filters the body's waste products into the urine. As indicated above (in the section on Goodpasture's syndrome), the possible effects of the damage caused by glomerulonephritis include the presence of white and red blood cells and excess protein in the urine, high blood pressure and extreme fatigue due to anaemia, if the damage becomes more permanent.

Other parts of the kidney that may be damaged following the deposition of antibodies/immune complexes include the tubules (which collect the urine filtered through the glomeruli and provide a conduit into the ureter, which in turn connects to the bladder) and the interstitium (the kidney tissue between the glomeruli and the tubules).

Most forms of glomerulonephritis (and other types of autoimmune kidney disease) require treatment with corticosteroids and other immuno-suppressive drugs.

Vasculitis

Vasculitis means inflammation of blood vessels. The definition implies that the blood vessels are the main site of the inflammation. As blood vessels supply every part of the body, clearly the consequences of inflammation will depend upon the location of the affected vessels.

Vasculitis may occur in patients with well-established autoimmune diseases such as systemic lupus erythematosus and rheumatoid arthritis, both discussed earlier in this chapter. However, at least seven different major types of vasculitis have been identified as distinct entities, namely:

- polyarteritis nodosa
- Wegener's granulomatosis
- Churg–Strauss vasculitis
- hypersensitivity vasculitis
- Henoch–Schönlein purpura
- giant cell arteritis
- Takayasu's arteritis

Several of these are named after the physicians who first described them. Although features such as fever and fatigue are common to most of these conditions, some, like giant cell arteritis and Takayasu's arteritis, tend to affect the larger arteries whilst polyarteritis nodosa affects the medium size vessels and Henoch–Schönlein purpura and hypersensitivity vasculitis affect small blood vessels (usually veins).

Polyarteritis nodosa

Most commonly affects males in middle age (40–60) causing kidney inflammation, joint pain, lung disease (coughing up blood, asthma) skin rashes, and inflammation of the nerves supplying the hands and feet.

Wegener's granulomatosis

Affects the sexes approximately equally, usually starting between the ages of 35 and 50. Among the common early features are stuffiness of the ear, nose, sinuses, and upper respiratory tract. Thus pain in the face and nosebleeds are frequent complaints. Subsequently kidney disease and inflammation of the joints, skin, and nervous system are common.

Churg–Strauss vasculitis

Much less common than Wegener's or polyarteritis nodosa, this condition is characterized by asthma, fever, swollen glands, heart failure, high blood pressure, and a large number of eosinophil cells in the blood.

Hypersensitivity vasculitis
The main feature of this condition is a florid skin rash in which the purple/blue, often slightly raised lumps may become necrotic and develop into ulcers. The rash may occur on its own but approximately half of the patients have joint pains, abdominal symptoms, fever, and fatigue.

Henoch–Schönlein purpura
This is a common childhood illness characterized by a red/purple rash especially on the legs, arthritis, abdominal pain, and kidney inflammation (in up to half the cases). The condition may also occur in adults.

Giant cell arteritis
This overlaps with another (more common) condition called polymyalgia rheumatica. Giant cell arteritis is found in the over 50s and is twice as common in women as in men. Headache, pain in the jaw on chewing and talking, scalp tenderness, fever, and fatigue are the major manifestations.

Takayasu's arteritis
This mainly occurs in women under 40 and living in Asia, Mexico, and the Far East. It causes a wide variety of symptoms including fever, weight loss, fatigue, headaches, aching of the arms during movement, and high blood pressure.

There are circumstantial reasons for placing these vasculitic conditions within the group of autoimmune diseases. Thus many, if not most, autoimmune diseases, e.g. lupus erythematosus, rheumatoid arthritis, and myositis may be complicated by vasculitis. Like patients with classic autoimmune diseases, those with vasculitis often require treatment with corticosteroids and other drugs to suppress the immune system. However, in the past few years more direct evidence has become available and it has been shown, at least for Wegener's, and to a lesser extent for polyarteritis nodosa, that fairly specific autoantibodies exist. Thus, in over 80 per cent of patients with Wegener's granulomatosis, antibodies to a component of the cytoplasm of neutrophils (known as cANCA) are present. These antibodies generally correspond with disease activity, and there is at least one claim that, in an animal model, these antibodies may be pathogenic.

Uveitis
The eye may sometimes be subject to autoimmune attack. In particular, uveitis can occur when the uvea—part of the covering layer of the eye—

is damaged by the immune system. The consequences of this damage are increased tear production, pain in the eye, decreased vision, and an intense dislike of bright light. The condition may require steroid treatment.

Inflammatory bowel disease

The causes of the inflammatory bowel diseases ulcerative colitis and Crohn's disease are uncertain, but there is some evidence to suggest that both are the result of an autoimmune attack.

Ulcerative colitis

Ulcerative colitis is limited to the large bowel or colon, and usually causes severe superficial inflammation of the lining or surface layer. It is associated with loose and often bloody motions. The affected colon is involved in a continuous manner. Women are a little more likely to get the disease and there is a tendency for it to run in some families. It appears to be very uncommon among Afro-Caribbean populations.

Crohn's disease

Crohn's disease may involve any portion of the alimentary tract from mouth to anus, but in a discontinuous fashion, i.e. healthy areas alternate with diseased sections. The inflammation is more deep-seated than in ulcerative colitis, with infiltration by lymphocytes, plasma cells, and other inflammatory cells. It mainly affects young adults and it also has a slight tendency to run in families.

Treatment

Both conditions may require steroid treatment, although certain sulphur-based drugs have been shown to be very helpful in the treatment of ulcerative colitis. Both diseases may be very severe and indeed life threatening.

Polyglandular syndrome

A small number of patients suffer from a curious autoimmune polyglandular syndrome. There are at least two types:

- The first damages the parathyroid and adrenal glands, causing hair loss, skin discoloration, and sometimes pernicious anaemia and chronic active hepatitis.
- The second type damages the adrenal glands and causes thyroid disease, frequently diabetes mellitus, pernicious anaemia, and chronic active hepatitis.

Antibodies may be found in the blood of either of these types of patients, who are very difficult to treat.

Links between autoimmune and infectious diseases

It is clear that there are intimate links between infectious agents and autoimmunity. In some cases the infectious agent may act as a trigger for an autoimmune condition, although only when the other factors—genetic, hormonal, dietary, etc.—are in place. Conversely, infectious diseases may cause certain autoimmune phenomena, by producing autoantibodies, without the development of symptoms and signs of infection.

A trigger?

Elsewhere in this book we suggest that infection due to a microbe (usually a virus or bacterium) may act as a trigger for an autoimmune disease in a patient in whom the other predisposing factors are present. Good examples of this phenomenon include diabetes mellitus and polymyositis, which have been shown to develop after infection with the Coxsackie virus. Many doctors who look after patients with systemic lupus erythematosus have observed that any kind of infection may cause a temporary flare-up in the patient's symptoms. Recently there have been attempts to link rheumatoid arthritis with bacterial infection by slow growing mycobacterium (a distant cousin of the bacterium that causes tuberculosis) or the bacterium *Proteus mirabilis*. Another, better established example, is the development of rheumatic fever after infection with streptococcal bacteria. In this condition, following exposure to the bacteria, which cause a sore throat and fever, the patient develops an irregular pulse and shortness of breath accompanied by a persistence of the fever. This condition occurs because the immune system, being unable to distinguish between the heart and some of the components of the invading bacteria, attacks the heart tissue.

Autoimmune features

Microbial infections, especially by viruses, may also give rise to a number of features that are often thought of as autoimmune. A good example of this is so-called 'reactive arthropathy', which occurs in individuals with a specific genetic marker on the surface of their cells. Following a gut infection, these patients may develop a variety of painful swollen joints. Similarly a condition called Reiter's syndrome is commonly observed following venereal exposure to the micro-organism *Chlamydia trachomatis*.

This is associated with a small number of painful swollen joints, inflammation of the urethra and conjunctiva, low back pain, and a rash on the soles of the feet. In these type of arthropathies it has proved difficult to identify the original infecting agent in the affected tissues. Furthermore, auto-antibodies are generally absent in these disorders.

Ankylosing spondylitis

A condition known as ankylosing spondylitis causes stiffness of the back starting in the sacroiliac joints at the base of the spine. This disease, most common in young men, has a striking genetic linkage as approximately 96 per cent of these patients carry the human leucocyte antigen B27 marker. It has been suggested that there is a similarity in structure between human leucocyte antigen B27 (present on cell surfaces) and a form of micro-organism known as *Klebsiella*. As *Klebsiella* is a bacterium, the body's immune system is primed to act against it. However, there is a danger that, after *Klebsiella* infection, this response will be triggered against anything looking like *Klebsiella*. If this similar structure is part of the body's own cells then there is a potential for self-damage.

Some studies have confirmed that patients with ankylosing spondylitis have increased amounts of *Klebsiella* organisms in their bowels. Thus it has been suggested that patients with ankylosing spondylitis are over-exposed to *Klebsiella* species that enter the body through the bowel wall. There are known to be special blood vessel connections between the bowel wall and the lower part of the spine close to where the disease begins. However, the precise mechanisms which lead to the development of the disease remain uncertain and some researchers give little credence to the '*Klebsiella* story'. Ankylosing spondylitis has no known cure but is treated symptomatically, with reasonable success in most cases, by non-steroidal anti-inflammatory drugs and physiotherapy.

AIDS

In recent years the acquired immune deficiency syndrome (AIDS) epidemic has been largely responsible for increasing our knowledge of the way in which the immune system functions. We know that AIDS is caused by a particular type of virus—a retrovirus known as the human immuno-deficiency virus (HIV). There is substantial evidence to suggest that human immunodeficiency virus can trigger a diverse range of autoimmune phenomena. For example, individuals infected with human immuno-deficiency virus and patients with AIDS have been known to develop Reiter's syndrome, lupus-like symptoms (including kidney inflammation, skin rash, and involvement of the nervous system), as well as some features reminiscent of polymyositis, Sjögren's syndrome, and rheumatoid arthritis. In addition, thyroid disease, multiple sclerosis, diabetes, and features of virtually all autoimmune disorders have been reported to occur.

Among the abnormalities found in the blood of AIDS patients are auto-antibodies that react with a variety of self-antigens, including the CD4+ helper T cells, which are largely destroyed during the course of the disease. Indeed, the presence of antilymphocyte autoantibodies has caused many investigators to speculate that in AIDS the immune system is destroyed by a civil war waged by elements of the immune system against one another.

Rubella

While the autoimmune aspect of AIDS is a recently recognized problem, a similar enigma associated with rubella (German measles) has been known for much longer. This virus can cause a transient arthritis in humans. Recently it has become clear that the virus may give rise to a disease that mimics rheumatoid arthritis. Thus patients may have swollen hands or even feet, early morning stiffness, and a feeling of tiredness. Fortunately, this is a short-lived disease that gets better on its own. It is as if the individual concerned does not have the ability to sustain a major attack on self-tissues, unlike patients who go on to develop 'true' auto-immune diseases, which often last for decades.

Epstein–Barr virus

Another virus that has excited great interest is the Epstein–Barr virus. This virus is associated with infectious mononucleosis (glandular fever), cancer of the nasopharynx (back of the throat), and a malignant tumour of lymphatic tissues known as Burkitt's lymphoma. There have also been suggestions that it may trigger rheumatoid arthritis. Immunologically, the virus is best known because it can infect and activate, in a random way, various B cells, and so cause antibody and autoantibody production.

Summary

The range of symptoms caused by autoimmune diseases is enormous. Nevertheless, the factors that combine to cause them are much the same and many of these conditions are treated with a small range of drugs that can suppress the immune system. These drugs do not, however, cure these diseases, and many have unpleasant side-effects. In the next chapter we review how some of these widely prescribed drugs work and some of the exciting developments in therapy.

6

Can anything be done once an autoimmune disease starts?

This century has witnessed dramatic advances in the treatment of autoimmune diseases. In some cases, identifying and supplying the 'missing' product of a gland destroyed by an autoimmune process has meant that the resulting disorder can be contained. Examples of this type of replacement are:

- the hormone thyroxine, which is no longer produced from the thyroid gland of patients with Hashimoto's thyroiditis;
- the hormone insulin, which the pancreas of patients with diabetes mellitus can no longer secrete.

The ability to transplant organs, such as the kidneys in patients with severe systemic lupus erythematosus, has also improved survival enormously. Most advances, however, relate to drug therapy. Many of the drugs currently available were introduced initially for the treatment of cancer. Although very helpful in controlling many autoimmune diseases they are not ideal because:

- as well as suppressing the abnormal parts of the immune system, other more normally functioning parts are suppressed and this increases the likelihood of infection;
- many are potentially toxic to the bone marrow;
- some, in large doses over long periods of time are linked to an increased risk of certain cancers.

Many new ideas are being explored but no cure for autoimmunity is on the immediate horizon.

Introduction

During the twentieth century diseases now known to be autoimmune have been treated with a wide variety of compounds from vitamin E to arsenic! Despite this treatment some patients did survive, but clearly more appropriate measures were required. In some cases, such as Hashimoto's thyroiditis (underactive thyroid) and diabetes mellitus, the ability to provide the missing hormone, thyroxine and insulin respectively, was the key to improving management. With other diseases serendipity played a major part in finding beneficial therapy. A good example was the introduction of gold treatment for rheumatoid arthritis. Gold injections were initially given because it was thought that the pathology of rheumatoid arthritis seen under the microscope resembled that of tuberculosis, which was at that time being treated by gold injections. Paradoxically it has since been established that gold treatment is of no value in tuberculosis but does have a useful part to play in controlling rheumatoid arthritis.

By the late 1940s, however, it became clear that it was going to be necessary to suppress the immune system in patients with autoimmune diseases, in order to bring these diseases under some form of control. Corticosteroids, which were introduced for treatment purposes at this time, were really a major breakthrough in this area. Subsequently a large number of other drugs which affect the functioning of the immune system have been introduced. Many, however, were initially used for the treatment of various forms of cancer. It must be emphasized that treatment with these drugs is no panacea, since many have side-effects which on occasion can be severe and even life-threatening. In this chapter the use of drugs now well established in the treatment of autoimmune diseases is considered together with some other treatment modalities. Less well established methods and more experimental procedures are also considered, since none of the longer established methods provides a cure and we are still seeking ways of stopping the destructive autoimmune process in its tracks and returning these rebel troops to their bases!

Well-established treatment

Corticosteroids

Short history

In April 1929 Philip Hench, an American physician working at the Mayo Clinic in the United States, observed a patient with rheumatoid arthritis, who had a remarkable remission during a bout of jaundice. During the next five years Dr Hench observed this phenomenon on many occasions and also noted a similar improvement in women with rheumatoid arthritis when they became pregnant. For several years he speculated whether an unknown factor might be responsible for the remission in pregnancy and during periods of jaundice. In September 1948, with the help of a colleague from the Department of Biochemistry at the Mayo Clinic, Dr Edward Kendal, Hench was able to administer a compound derived from bile (a fluid secreted by the liver) to a volunteer patient with rheumatoid arthritis. The effect was described later by Dr Hench as 'unlike that of any previous remedy or of any condition, except pregnancy or jaundice'. The active component which had been given to the patient was a form of corticosteroid.

Within a few months a drug company (Armour Laboratories) was able to provide Dr Hench with another hormone that had been isolated from the pituitary gland. This hormone, known as adrenocorticotrophic hormone (ACTH) is usually released from the pituitary gland in the brain (see Figure 6.1) and acts on the adrenal gland (situated just on top of the kidneys) to stimulate the production of various steroid hormones.

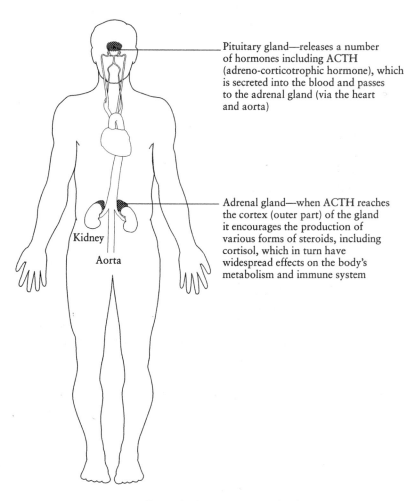

Pituitary gland—releases a number of hormones including ACTH (adreno-corticotrophic hormone), which is secreted into the blood and passes to the adrenal gland (via the heart and aorta)

Adrenal gland—when ACTH reaches the cortex (outer part) of the gland it encourages the production of various forms of steroids, including cortisol, which in turn have widespread effects on the body's metabolism and immune system

Kidney

Aorta

Figure 6.1 Effects of adrenocorticotrophic hormone.

A film of the first patient injected with adrenocorticotrophic hormone is quite remarkable. A middle-aged woman with rheumatoid arthritis, obviously in severe pain and with marked swelling of many of her joints, is shown trying to climb over a small set of steps. This she does with great difficulty. After a series of adrenocorticotrophic hormone injections over the next few weeks, she was again asked to climb the steps. This time she ran quickly up and down them. The drug was stopped and, a month later, the patient was again asked to climb the steps. She is shown to be back at square one, barely able to crawl over the steps.

Over the past 40 years major attempts to work out the beneficial effects of corticosteroids have been made. It is now clear that these effects are multiple and complex. The major actions of these drugs are:

- Anti-inflammatory effects:
  —a fall in the numbers of blood lymphocytes (especially T helper cells);
  —a fall in the numbers of blood monocytes and eosinophils;
  —altered functioning of monocytes and neutrophils limiting their ability to take part in immune and inflammatory processes;
  —reduction in the release of cytokines from monocytes, macrophages, and lymphocytes;
  —some reduction in immunoglobulin production;
  —block the release of potentially harmful enzymes by neutrophils.
- Increase in protein metabolism.
- Block some actions of insulin.
- Some anti-allergic properties.

Side-effects of corticosteroids

Early reports about the beneficial effects of steroids in a range of diseases, from hay fever to systemic lupus erythematosus, became known very quickly. Steroids very often have a rapid effect, improving the general state and the feeling of well-being of a patient. There is no doubt that they have saved the lives of many patients who might have died from conditions such as systemic lupus erythematosus, autoimmune haemolytic anaemia, thrombocytopenia, myositis, and vasculitis. There is, however, a potential price to pay for these benefits. Gradually, the unpleasant side-effects of the corticosteroid drugs became obvious; the most common of which are:

- weight gain;
- high blood pressure;
- thinning of the bones (osteoporosis);
- increased risk of diabetes;

- increased risk of infection;
- change in body shape—thin arms and legs, increase in the size of the abdomen;
- poor sleep (insomnia);
- increase in abdominal stretch marks, often with a blue colour.

In a general sense, the higher the dose of steroids and the longer they are prescribed, the greater the risk of side-effects. However, it is not possible to say in advance precisely what constitutes too much steroid for any individual, as the variation in response is very wide.

Administration of corticosteroids

Although corticosteroids can be administered by intramuscular or intravenous injection, they are usually given by mouth. With experience it has become possible to minimize the likelihood of side-effects by constantly trying to prescribe the lowest effective dose of steroids, and for the shortest possible time. However, it is common, when treating many of the severe types of autoimmune diseases, to use relatively large doses of steroids in the short term and then reduce the dose as quickly as possible—this also minimizes the chance of developing side-effects. The major indications for the use of corticosteroids in autoimmune diseases are shown below.

It is possible that giving steroids on alternate days, for example giving 30 mg on one day and none the next day (as opposed to giving 15 mg on each day), might also help to reduce the side-effects. Some patients find this difficult to manage and prefer to take the same dose each day. However, in the case of a flare-up of disease symptoms, for example in rheumatoid arthritis, there may be an advantage in giving a large intramuscular dose of steroid, which often benefits the patient for several weeks, or even months. Table 1 indicates the main uses of corticosteroids.

Intravenous injection

Intravenous injection gives more immediate access to the immune system than taking steroids by mouth or intramuscular injection. Many studies have shown the effects on the immune system of large doses of steroids given by intravenous injection. In fact, most of the effects are reversed within 48 hours, although some can last for several weeks. Intravenous corticosteroids are still used in severe cases of lupus when the disease is very active.

Although corticosteroids are useful in a wide range of autoimmune diseases, they are of no real use in diabetes mellitus, Hashimoto's thyroiditis,

Table 1 Main uses of corticosteroids.

Disease	Potential value
Diseases with limited organ involvement	
Autoimmune haemolytic anaemia	High doses of corticosteroids will frequently arrest the disease and help to increase the haemoglobin level (other drugs may be required).
Autoimmune thrombocytopenia	High doses of corticosteroids are invariably needed to control the disease and boost the level of platelets (other drugs may be required).
Chronic active hepatitis	Steroids are often effective in controlling, if not curing, the symptoms of liver damage.
Pemphigus	Virtually always requires steroids to control symptoms (other drugs may be required).
Myositis	About 80% of patients with myositis of the muscles show some response to steroids. Even with the help of other drugs, over one-third of patients remain weak after several years.
Myasthenia gravis	Steroids are required occasionally for severe cases
Multiple sclerosis	Use of steroids is debated. They may help to shorten an acute attack but their long-term use is rarely of much benefit.
Diseases affecting many organs	
Systemic lupus erythematosus	Steroids are widely used to control the effects on the lungs, heart, kidney, blood cells, and central nervous system. They are usually required for months or years and may need to be supplemented by other drugs in really severe cases.
Sjögren's syndrome	Steroids are occasionally required in cases associated with severe swelling of the parotid glands.
Rheumatoid arthritis	Many victims are middle-aged women already predisposed to osteoporosis. Steroids are difficult to stop and so many rheumatologists now try to avoid using steroids by mouth for these patients. However, steroids are useful in reducing joint inflammation and around one-third of patients are taking them at any one time. Occasionally steroid injections into the joints can be helpful and an intramuscular 'shot' of steroids will often help bring a relapse under control.
Scleroderma	Steroids are of limited use in the early stages of the disease only.
Vasculitis	Steroids are often used, though some antimalarial drugs are helpful. Steroids often need to be supplemented with other drugs to suppress the immune system.

Graves' disease, and primary biliary cirrhosis. In contrast, patients with conditions that are not necessarily autoimmune in origin, such as asthma, often benefit from steroids. In the case of asthma, steroids may be given as a form of aerosol and are 'squirted' into the bronchial passages.

Immunosuppressive (cytotoxic) drugs

Cytotoxic drugs are designed to kill those cells in the immune system thought to be responsible for causing autoimmune disease. However, the drugs are not selectively toxic for these cells, but can kill any cell, especially those that divide and multiply rapidly. This is why nausea, vomiting, and diarrhoea are common side-effects—the cells in the lining of the gut are among the most rapidly dividing in the body. The ability of a cytotoxic drug to reduce the number of immunologically reactive cells depends upon several interlinked factors, including:

- the frequency with which the target cell is dividing;
- the precise phase of the cell's reproductive cycle in which a particular drug exerts its toxic effect.

Many immunosuppressive or cytotoxic drugs are used to treat severe cases of autoimmune diseases. Most of these drugs were introduced originally to treat cancer, and it was only later that their use in the treatment of autoimmunity was appreciated. A guide to these drugs, indicating how they work, for which conditions they are used, and their side-effects is given in Table 2 (see page 114).

Anticancer drugs

The first anticancer drug to be shown to have major suppressive effects on the immune system was 6-mercaptopurine. Studies of this drug in the late 1950s by Robert Schwartz and William Dameshek in Boston were a real landmark. Within four years Roy Calne in England showed that this drug and its derivative azathioprine were successful in prolonging survival of kidney grafts in the dog. By the late 1960s the combination of corticosteroids and azathioprine had been shown to be an effective regime for increasing the chance of a successful organ transplant in human beings. It has only been in the last few years that this combination has been replaced in some cases by the new drug cyclosporin which is discussed later on page 115. Other powerful drugs used initially for treating patients with cancer and now widely used in the treatment of autoimmune diseases are cyclophosphamide, methotrexate, and chlorambucil. Table 2 provides information about the mechanism(s) by which they work, the diseases they are prescribed for, and their major side-effects.

Table 2 Immunosuppressive drugs used in the treatment of autoimmune disease.

Drug	How does it work?	When is it used?	Side-effects
Azathioprine	Blocks the synthesis of compounds used by the body to make DNA. This reduces the rate at which cells multiply.	Widely used to stop the rejection of organ transplants. Also used in systemic lupus erythematosus (SLE), rheumatoid arthritis, myositis, chronic active hepatitis, autoimmune haemolytic anaemia and thrombocytopenia, and myasthenia gravis.	Skin rashes, diarrhoea, nausea, and vomiting (occasionally). Occasionally results in cessation of the bone marrow function, resulting in anaemia and low levels of white blood cells and platelets.
Cyclophosphamide	Cross-links DNA strands, resulting in immediate death of some cells and death during cell division of others. The effect on B cells is more severe than the effect on the T cells.	Kidney and some neurological disease in SLE, some cases of rheumatoid arthritis (if there is vasculitis) and in some cases of autoimmune thrombocytopenia/anaemia showing little response to steroids alone.	Hair loss, nausea, and vomiting can be severe. Infertility may occur and the effects on the bone marrow are as with azathioprine. Cystitis with blood in the urine can also occur.
Methotrexate	Blocks an enzyme that is involved in the production of DNA.	Now widely used in the treatment of rheumatoid arthritis and patients with psoriasis who also get arthritis; used much less frequently in SLE or myositis.	Nausea, vomiting, diarrhoea, and anaemia, bone marrow suppression, causing the problems seen with azathioprine. Liver damage also occurs.
Chlorambucil	As for cyclophosphamide.	The least frequently used cytotoxic drug. Occasionally used in SLE, rheumatoid arthritis, and Waldenström's macro-globulinaemia. More widely used for certain types of lymphomas and leukaemias.	Occasional skin rashes, nausea, vomiting, diarrhoea, bone marrow suppression, as with azathioprine. Increased production of fibrous tissue in the lungs is a rare but serious problem.

Side-effects

As well as those side-effects shown on page 114, there is an increased, although small, risk of cancer in autoimmune patients treated with these agents. This is ironic, given the fact that the drugs were introduced originally to treat cancer! Furthermore, there is a greatly increased risk of tumours of the skin, lymphomas, and occasionally leukaemias, in transplant patients receiving immunosuppressive drugs—up to 100 times that of individuals not taking the drug.

Cyclosporin A

Cyclosporin A was discovered in 1972. It is produced from two types of fungi and has been shown to have a variety of effects on the immune system, most importantly, the ability to suppress many actions of the T cells. It thus acts to prevent the rejection of a transplanted organ. It has proved very useful and is often prescribed concurrently with steroids and azathioprine or instead of them.

In the past 15 years, cyclosporin A has been used to treat virtually every single autoimmune disease. Perhaps its greatest use has been in the treatment of diabetes mellitus. Provided that it can be given early enough in the course of diabetes, it may be possible to avoid having to use insulin at all and, if insulin is needed, it is in smaller doses than would have been the case without the drug.

Side-effects

As with all drugs, an important limitation on its use has been the side-effects it can induce. In the case of cyclosporin these include damage to the kidneys, development of lymphomas, a tendency to an increase in body hair, and severe nausea.

How does it work?

The mechanism by which cyclosporin acts in autoimmune diseases is only partially understood. One current view is that it inhibits immune responses that require T cell help by inhibiting the production of cytokines. However, a host of other possible mechanisms have been suggested and the situation remains to be clarified.

Plasma exchange

The idea behind plasma exchange (plasmapheresis) is relatively simple (see Figure 6.2). Whole blood is removed from a patient's vein and passed into

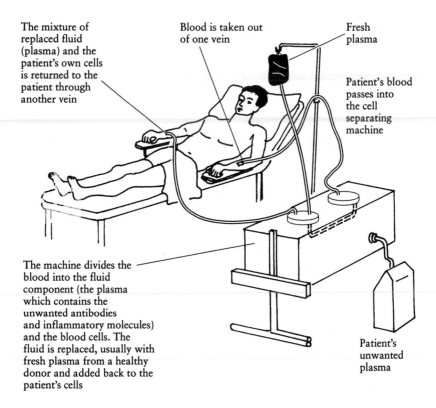

The mixture of replaced fluid (plasma) and the patient's own cells is returned to the patient through another vein

Blood is taken out of one vein

Fresh plasma

Patient's blood passes into the cell separating machine

The machine divides the blood into the fluid component (the plasma which contains the unwanted antibodies and inflammatory molecules) and the blood cells. The fluid is replaced, usually with fresh plasma from a healthy donor and added back to the patient's cells

Patient's unwanted plasma

Figure 6.2 Plasma exchange.

a machine that separates the cells in the blood from the fluid (plasma). The patient's plasma, which will contain immune complexes and/or other harmful factors that are involved in the autoimmune disease process, is discarded and replaced by fresh plasma from healthy individuals. The healthy plasma is mixed with the patient's own blood cells in the machine and the newly reconstructed blood is then passed back into the patient's body.

Although plasma exchange was very popular in the late 1970s and early 1980s, it has only been shown to benefit a small number of diseases. Plasma exchange was first tried successfully in macroglobulinaemia and multiple myeloma—cancers that cause a great increase in the numbers of antibodies in the blood. It is also effective for patients with Goodpasture's syndrome and myasthenia gravis.

Plasma exchange has had variable results in other autoimmune diseases. In polymyositis there has been only one report strongly commending its use. However, a recent study of 11 patients with Graves' disease with severe eye involvement supported the view that intensive plasma exchange followed by treatment with immunosuppressive drugs was useful. In contrast, although there are case reports describing dramatic improvement in some patients with systemic lupus erythematosus, in the main few patients derive much benefit from plasma exchange.

On balance, plasma exchange is now thought to have little part to play in the treatment of autoimmune diseases—a conclusion based on its marginal clinical benefit in the majority of cases and the fact that it is extremely expensive.

It is possible to be even more selective about the type of substance removed from the blood. Thus lymphophoresis—the removal of the lymphoid cells—can be undertaken. This procedure has been shown to be of modest short-term use in the treatment of rheumatoid arthritis. Not surprisingly it tends to be reserved for the more severe cases, but even here its role remains somewhat controversial.

Total lymph node irradiation

This technique, developed more than 20 years ago, uses radiation directed at lymphoid tissues; other body tissues are shielded by lead to prevent damage. X-rays are thus targeted at the lymph nodes found in the neck, thorax, abdomen, and groin. Most lymphocytes are very sensitive and easily damaged by X-rays. Radiation causes a major reduction in the numbers of lymphocytes in lymphoid organs (liver and spleen) and suppresses the normal functioning of many cells.

Like immunosuppressive drugs, total lymph node irradiation was first introduced for the treatment of cancer, notably for tumours of the lymphoid cells. It was soon realized, however, that the treatment affected the immune system:

● It reduces the number of lymphocytes in the blood.
● It alters the immune system's interactions and responses to antigens.

Once the treatment has ceased, the numbers of lymphocytes in the blood gradually return to normal over 1 or 2 years. Curiously, however, on recovery the majority of the lymphocytes are B cells—the effect on the T cells seems to be longer-lasting. Furthermore, among the T cells, it is the helper cells that are particularly affected.

Side-effects

The most common side-effects of total lymph node irradiation therapy are:

● fatigue;

- loss of appetite;
- diarrhoea;
- weight loss;
- occasional infection with shingles.

Sterility is an inevitable consequence when the ovaries are irradiated, although this complication can be prevented by first surgically relocating the ovaries to a position where they can be more easily shielded during treatment.

If the thyroid is not shielded, approximately 20 per cent of patients will develop underactivity of the thyroid gland (hypothyroidism) and are also probably at an increased risk of thyroid cancer.

Severe complications can sometimes occur:

- suppression of the bone marrow cells;
- chronic inflammation of the lung tissue;
- inflammation of the heart;
- severe viral or bacterial infections.

The most feared complication of total lymphoid radiation—the development of tumours—was found to occur very rarely in over 3000 patients with Hodgkin's disease (a type of cancer) who were followed up for 10 years after completion of treatment.

Total lymph node irradiation is thus a powerful immunosuppressive type of treatment—it produces its effects by altering the functioning of T cells and appears to target the T helper cells. It can induce long-term remissions in established autoimmune diseases but it may cause serious side-effects—nausea, vomiting, increased risk of infections, and a reduced ability of the bone marrow to generate new blood cells. All of these problems, together with the slight risk of tumours developing, greatly restrict its use. At the moment, therefore, this type of therapy is restricted to those better able to tolerate it (i.e. individuals under 50 years of age and in good general health) who have severe disease, notably lupus or rheumatoid arthritis, for whom other forms of therapy have not been beneficial.

Less well established and experimental treatment

Dietary manipulation

Altering the diet as a way of helping to treat autoimmune diseases has attracted much interest in the last decade. Diet therapy for rheumatoid arthritis, multiple sclerosis, and systemic lupus erythematosus has attracted particular attention.

Diet treatment takes several forms:

- The total calorie intake can be reduced.
- The balance of the diet can be altered, so that, for example, the amount of fat is reduced but total calorie intake is maintained by increasing the amount of protein and carbohydrate.
- Supplements may be added, notably various forms of fish oil.

Reduced calorie intake

So far, very few experiments of reduced calorie consumption have been conducted in patients with autoimmune diseases. A trial in patients with rheumatoid arthritis showed that fasting was accompanied by a reduction in joint pain, stiffness, and medication requirements. However, the study was not well controlled. There has also been a claim that some symptoms of rheumatoid arthritis can be improved by a vegetarian diet.

As with all attempts at nutritional manipulation, the most difficult problem is persuading patients to stick rigidly to a diet. Experience confirms that even individuals who are obese and desperately want to lose weight find that maintaining a low calorie diet, which would clearly be beneficial, can be very difficult.

Altering the balance

Restricting fats

The effects of fat intake have been examined in some detail in the last 10 years, not only the total amount of fat ingested, but also the particular types of fat (notably saturated or unsaturated fat). It is thought that the influence of fat on autoimmunity depends on the synthesis of prostaglandins and leucotrienes, which have various effects on the immune system (as discussed in Chapter 3). These chemicals are manufactured from arachidonic acid and the absence of this in the diet of has been shown to improve survival in various animal models of autoimmune diseases.

A recent study from the USA has shown that fish oils containing long chain highly polyunsaturated fatty acids may help a wide variety of diseases, including rheumatoid arthritis. Similarly, in systemic lupus erythematosus, a recent study in which patients had their total fat intake reduced to 25 per cent or less of the total dietary calories (in most Western diets it constitutes over 30 per cent) with a fish oil supplement, improved the outcome over a 3-month period.

The rationale behind supplementing the diet with fish and other oils is that high levels of certain polyunsaturated fatty acids change the balance of leucotrienes and prostaglandins and produce a more balanced and less inflammatory state.

Restricting protein

Few studies have looked at protein restriction but those that have found that diets low in certain amino acids, as well as diets supplemented with particular synthetic amino acids, have all tended to prolong the survival and decrease the numbers of autoantibodies.

Restricting vitamins

There is some evidence that vitamins may play a role in influencing autoimmunity. For example, a diet deficient in vitamin A has been shown to aggravate autoimmunity. A vitamin E-enriched diet has been claimed to induce remissions in patients with lupus, scleroderma, and myositis, although the evidence of these studies must be regarded as provisional.

Interest in vitamin C was sparked a few years ago when it was claimed that large doses were the answer to many ailments, including the common cold and cancer. These views have not gained widespread support and there is really no compelling evidence to suggest that vitamin C therapy has a useful role to play in the treatment of autoimmune disease.

Restricting minerals

The effects of minerals are not particularly well researched but zinc deficiency has been shown to delay the onset of autoimmune manifestations in lupus-prone mice and supplementing the diet with selenium improved the survival.

Supplementation

Dietary regulation, particularly a low fat diet or fish oil supplementation, appears to be useful in the management of some autoimmune diseases. Supplementation of the diet with evening primrose oil and various fish oils has also provided some promising results to date. Studies carried out in Glasgow on rheumatoid arthritis patients have shown that evening primrose oil alone, or the combination of evening primrose oil and fish oil, can produce transient clinical improvement and, in some cases, reduce the need for anti-inflammatory drugs. However, it is doubtful whether these dietary supplements can modify the disease in the longer term.

A recent report from the USA has suggested that supplementing the diet of patients with rheumatoid arthritis with (chicken) collagen may also be beneficial. The mechanism by which this approach might be working is known as 'oral tolerization'. This process aims to take advantage of a trick used by the normal immune system to prevent an immune reaction to food. Foreign proteins entering the body in food pass through the digestive system, which is able to suppress an immune response to these proteins instead of triggering one. Oral tolerization attempts to reduce or minimize autoimmune attacks by feeding the patients forms of protein (collagen, in the case of rheumatoid arthritis) that are found at the site of autoimmune disease and might have triggered the autoimmune attack in the first place.

A general strategy which the above approach utilizes is based on the accurate identification of self-antigens which form the target of an auto-immune attack. The theory suggests that exposing the immune system to some form of such a self-antigen by an alternative route will allow the immune system to become tolerant of the self-antigen. To continue the military metaphor used elsewhere in the book, this additional self-antigen draws the fire of the immune attack allowing the bulk of the self-antigen elsewhere in the body to remain unharmed.

Apart from the example of feeding collagen to patients with rheumatoid arthritis, this approach has been studied in experimental autoimmune encephalomyelitis, adjuvant arthritis, and diabetes in non-obese diabetic mice. In the main the methods have consisted of providing suitable self-antigens by mouth.

If patients are prepared to undertake lengthy periods of dietary change there may well be advantages in terms of a general reduction in their symptoms and requirement for the drugs they need to control their disease. It is very unlikely, given the multiple factors involved in the cause of these autoimmune diseases, that dietary manipulation alone will cure any of them.

Hormonal manipulation

The increased frequency with which women suffer from autoimmune diseases is very striking. Given this, it is not surprising that attempts have been made to treat these disorders with sex hormones.

The use of sex hormones in autoimmune diseases has not been extensive. One particular drug—danazol (a male sex hormone)—has been studied in various conditions. One of the great problems of prescribing a male hormone to women is that the side-effects (the appearance of masculine features such as deepening of the voice, increasing muscles, and an increase in body hair) are unacceptable to most women. The attraction of danazol has been that these side-effects are minimal. The drug has been used in patients with systemic lupus erythematosus and in haemolytic anaemia and thrombocytopenia. However, only a small number of patients appear to benefit—usually transiently—and, to date, danazol has not found widespread acceptance as a useful treatment. Nevertheless, the notion that altering the balance of hormones within the body might lessen the impact of a major autoimmune attack remains attractive. Several other drugs, which are thought to have these effects, are currently under investigation.

Antibodies to the human leucocyte antigens

Most autoimmune diseases have been shown to be linked to the human leucocyte antigens, which are concerned with regulating the responses of the immune system (see Chapter 3). These molecules are situated on the surface of cells that present antigen to the T cells. The human leucocyte antigen and the processed antigen are closely associated and together bind to the T cell receptors.

The exact manner in which a particular human leucocyte antigen contributes to the development of an autoimmune disease remains uncertain. Nevertheless many research groups have attempted to manipulate these human leucocyte antigens on the grounds that this would in some way alter the immune response and thus may also alter the process of the autoimmune disease.

Most of the experiments to date have focused on treatment with specially prepared antibodies—monoclonal antibodies (see Figure 6.3)—which are directed against the major histocompatibility complex molecules. Monoclonal antibodies are antibodies from a single type or clone of cell. The generation and isolation of monoclonal antibodies has revolutionized immunology over the last 15 years. They are widely used in therapeutic and diagnostic applications, and are also a tool for basic research.

For obvious reasons, most of the experiments to date have been undertaken in mouse models of autoimmune diseases and in the main have focused on treating the animals concerned with monoclonal antibodies, directed against the product of major histocompatibility complex genes. Among the autoimmune models studied are experimental allergic encephalitis, a model for multiple sclerosis, the lupus-like disease in mice, experimental autoimmune thyroiditis, experimental autoimmune uveitis (an eye disease), collagen-induced arthritis, and experimental myasthenia gravis.

The precise mechanism of action of the monoclonal antibodies remains

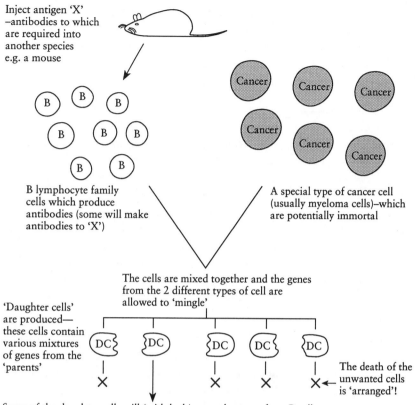

Inject antigen 'X' –antibodies to which are required into another species e.g. a mouse

B lymphocyte family cells which produce antibodies (some will make antibodies to 'X')

A special type of cancer cell (usually myeloma cells)–which are potentially immortal

The cells are mixed together and the genes from the 2 different types of cell are allowed to 'mingle'

'Daughter cells' are produced— these cells contain various mixtures of genes from the 'parents'

The death of the unwanted cells is 'arranged'!

Some of the daughter cells will (with luck) carry the genes from B cells which allow them to make antibodies to 'X' and the genes from the cancer cell which make them potentially immortal. Thus one clone of cells is produced which in theory could go on making anti-DNA antibodies forever

Figure 6.3 Making monoclonal antibodies.

unclear, and probably varies according to the target each individual antibody recognizes. Some, it is thought, might influence the ability of the T cells to bind to the complex of antigen and human leucocyte antigen. There is limited evidence that monoclonal antibodies trigger the production of suppressive T cells, which would depress the local active autoimmune disease. They also seem to have a more direct effect on B cells, the numbers of which tend to decrease following this type of therapy.

An obstacle to using this type of monoclonal antibody therapy has been the finding that it can cause an unexpected blood clotting problem. More work remains to be done before this type of approach can be considered seriously for treatment. In contrast, monoclonal antibody therapy to one of the major chemical messengers involved in inflammation—TNFalpha— has been used successfully in rheumatoid arthritis. The studies to date are short term, but do seem encouraging.

Anti-T cell receptor treatment and T cell vaccination

T cell receptors are intimately involved in the handling of antigens (see Chapter 3 for details). Like antibodies, T cell receptors have many different shapes, so that they can recognize many different antigens, and vary considerably from one individual to another. Researchers are now trying to determine whether there is restricted use of T cell receptors in auto-immune disease. The hope is that if a limited subpopulation of T cells involved in a given disease can be identified, then a therapeutic strategy based on the recognition and elimination of the offending cells can be developed. Indeed, some evidence of a limited repertoire of T cell receptor usage has been demonstrated in multiple sclerosis, rheumatoid arthritis, and thyroiditis. Acting on this information, two types of treatment strategies are currently being developed:

1. *Passive therapy with monoclonal antibodies.* A T cell with a distinct disease-associated receptor can be used to generate monoclonal anti-bodies. Once made, the antibodies are injected into the patient's blood-stream and the T cells in question are eliminated.

2. *Active therapy or vaccination of the patient with a small, unique, portion of the receptor molecule.* This strategy is complex because not only does a pathogenic T cell need to be cloned (i.e. isolated then produced in large numbers), but its receptor needs to be analysed in detail after which small protein fragments from it must be synthesized and tested. The T cell receptor fragments are injected in small quanti-ties into the patient (unlike the passive therapy, where relatively large quantities of the monoclonal antibody are injected directly into the blood) with the intent that the individual will generate an antibody response against the disease-associated T cells.

The concept of vaccination against autoimmune disease is extremely attractive and warrants vigorous investigation.

Manipulation of the idiotype network

As described in Chapter 2, antibodies contain sections that are relatively similar (the Fc region) and other sections that are very variable and specific to particular antigens (the Fab regions). The variability is brought about by differences in the amino acids that make up the Fab region of the antibody. This great variation means that the immune system can recognize the many different forms and shapes taken by foreign bacteria, viruses, and other external threats. Unfortunately the variation in these Fab regions (portions of which are known as idiotypes) is such that the immune system frequently regards them as akin to foreign material and makes antibodies (anti-idiotypes) against the variable Fab regions.

Certain idiotypes seem to be associated with disease. For example, antibodies carrying particular idiotypes are frequently found in the kidneys and skin biopsies of patients with systemic lupus erythematosus. A theory has been developed suggesting that blocking a potentially harmful idiotype with an anti-idiotype antibody might be beneficial. Four types of therapeutic strategies relating to this approach are shown in Figure 6.4 and detailed below:

1. Anti-DNA antibodies carrying a potentially harmful idiotype are injected. The idea is that the body will make an anti-idiotypic antibody that will shut down the production of anti-DNA antibodies. This experiment worked very well but only for a short period of time. Eventually anti-DNA autoantibodies carrying different pathogenic idiotypes were produced.

2. An anti-idiotypic antibody was injected to block the anti-DNA antibodies carrying the pathogenic idiotype. This approach had transient success but eventually the mechanisms driving the disease escaped the control of the therapeutic antibody.

3. The anti-idiotypic antibody was in a sense used as a guided missile— it identified antibodies carrying the idiotype and cells producing such antibodies but, because the anti-idiotype was tagged to a toxic drug, the cell producing the harmful autoantibodies was destroyed.

4. A variant of plasma exchange was used, in which the plasma of the patients with lupus was separated by a plasma exchange machine and then passed down a column of material containing the anti-idiotypic antibody. In theory, this column would retain any autoantibodies bearing the common idiotype, while other plasma components were allowed through and passed back into the patient. The final results of the study are still awaited.

High dose intravenous gammaglobulin

There has been growing interest over the past five years in the possible benefit of intravenous high dose gammaglobulins, which have been prepared from the plasma of healthy individuals.

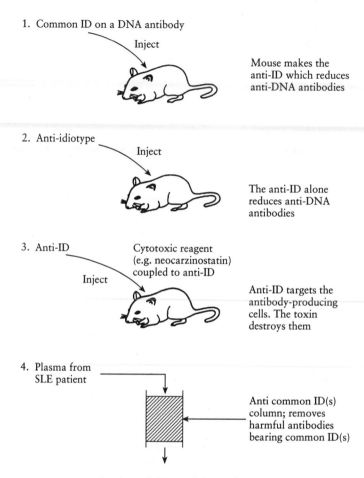

1. Common ID on a DNA antibody

   Inject

   Mouse makes the anti-ID which reduces anti-DNA antibodies

2. Anti-idiotype

   Inject

   The anti-ID alone reduces anti-DNA antibodies

3. Anti-ID

   Cytotoxic reagent (e.g. neocarzinostatin) coupled to anti-ID

   Inject

   Anti-ID targets the antibody-producing cells. The toxin destroys them

4. Plasma from SLE patient

   Anti common ID(s) column; removes harmful antibodies bearing common ID(s)

Figure 6.4 Idiotype (ID)/anti-idiotype therapeutic strategies.

Most experience with high dose intravenous gammaglobulin in children has been gained in chronic idiopathic thrombocytopenic purpura (which causes a low platelet count and a tendency to bleed). The alternative treatment to this type of therapy is surgical removal of the spleen and it has been estimated that intravenous gammaglobulin may avoid this major operation in about 50 per cent of patients. Adults with this form of purpura may also respond to high dose intravenous gammaglobulin, although with fewer long-term successes.

Myasthenia gravis has also been treated successfully for a short period with high dose intravenous gammaglobulin, with major clinical improvement beginning 3 to 6 days after therapy. A recent report has also described some success in treating patients with myositis by this method.

Mode of action

Much has been written about the potential modes of action of this form of treatment. It has been suggested that the therapeutic gammaglobulins may contain a large number of anti-idiotype antibodies, which help to shut down the production of, or at least block the effects of, antibodies that cause the disease. Other theories suggest that:

- Intravenous gammaglobulin affects T cell populations, causing an increase in T suppressor cell activity, and thus reducing the number of antibodies produced by B cells.
- Suppression of antiplatelet antibody synthesis occurs in patients with thrombocytopenia.
- Intravenous gammaglobulin blocks certain receptors on the surface of phagocytic cells in the circulation and this causes the reduction in self-destructive activity in the immune system.

Clonal deletion therapy

An attractive alternative to drugs that suppress the immune system in a random way is to try to destroy or suppress those particular lymphocytes that are responsible for producing autoantibodies. Two strategies have been developed:

1. antibodies that bind directly to T cells and block their effects;
2. toxins are linked to various self-antigens in the hope of killing the lymphocytes that are inclined to bind to them.

An example of the first strategy is the use of monoclonal antibodies directed against T helper cells bearing the CD4 marker. Preliminary studies have shown promising results in the treatment of rheumatoid arthritis. Long-term clinical trials continue.

The second strategy requires the administration of toxins bound to self-antigens. The use of this type of 'immunological bullet' requires the antigen to be identified and purified. One animal model in which this prerequisite has been met is experimental allergic encephalitis (a form of myasthenia gravis). Pretreatment of the acetylcholine receptor (which is the target for attack in this autoimmune condition) linked with a toxin was shown to selectively eliminate harmful cells within the immune system. In another experiment a toxin called ricin was linked to thyroglobulin, a normal component of the thyroid gland. It was shown that the abnormal functioning of lymphocytes from patients with Hashimoto's thyroiditis treated with this 'immunotoxin' was significantly blocked. The levels of the antibodies to thyroglobulin were also reduced significantly. This strategy requires a very fine balance of toxin and self-antigen, as the deleterious effects of the toxin could easily become evident.

Treatment with interferon

Interferon is one of the chemical messengers described in detail in Chapter 2. A limited number of studies have attempted to find our whether interferon might have a useful role to play in the treatment of autoimmune conditions. Studies in the early 1980s showed that when alpha and gamma interferon were injected into lupus-prone mice the manifestations of the disease increased and the life span of the animals was considerably reduced. Indeed, even genetically normal mice, when exposed to interferon directly or indirectly, were shown to develop inflammation of the kidney. Perhaps a little surprisingly, this form of treatment has been used for some human conditions. For example a rare disease called mixed cryoglobulineamia (associated with the precipitation of particular types of protein in the cold) when treated with interferon alpha, was shown to respond very successfully, with very few side-effects. There are several theories as to precisely why this treatment might work, including the possible restoration of normal control of B cells through the effect on the function of T cell and natural killer cells.

Interferons may also have beneficial effects on rheumatoid arthritis. It is thought that interferon gamma can block the effects of another cytokine, interleukin-4 (IL4), and B lymphocyte growth, consequently reducing the level of various autoantibodies including rheumatoid factor. As implied earlier, however, other actions of interferon might exacerbate certain diseases. For example, it was shown that exposure of certain cells from the synovium of patients with rheumatoid arthritis to gamma interferon led to their multiplication. There are also recent reports that interferon alpha used in the treatment of some forms of leukaemia may cause the development of antibodies to DNA and thyroid antigens.

Other forms of treatment

The intractable nature of many autoimmune diseases, coupled with the side-effects of conventional therapy, have led to innumerable therapeutic approaches, often based on the slimmest of evidence. However, recent attempts to treat rheumatoid arthritis with antibiotics, and especially antimycobacterial drugs, have stimulated some interest. Indeed, there is growing evidence that exposure to some, almost certainly very slow-growing, form of mycobacterium plays a part in the origin of rheumatoid arthritis. In the United States, antibiotic therapy, notably using tetracycline, is being used in the treatment of rheumatoid arthritis, although more studies are needed. There has also been considerable interest in the use of drugs usually prescribed for the treatment of tuberculosis for patients with rheumatoid arthritis. However, despite some early claims of success, a recent study published in the *British Journal of Rheumatology* gives rather scant support to this approach. However, it must be remembered that the drug used—rifampicin—may simply be the wrong drug.

GLOSSARY

Acetylcholine/acetylcholine receptor: Acetylcholine is a chemical messenger. It is released from the end of a nerve after the nerve has been stimulated. It crosses the small gap between the nerve and the adjacent muscle fibres, where it attaches to a component of the muscle fibre (the receptor) and causes the muscle fibre to twitch.

Addison's disease: Insufficiency of the **adrenal glands** causing low blood pressure, anaemia, salt loss but potassium retention, and increased skin pigmentation.

Adhesion molecules: Found mainly on lymphocyte cells, they consist of a number of surface proteins and carbohydrates that help to give the various white cell populations their different properties.

Adrenal gland: Situated just above the kidney the adrenal gland is subdivided into the outer layer, or cortex, and the inner medulla. The gland is responsible for the production of a variety of hormones including some sex hormones and corticosteroids.

Adrenocorticotrophic hormone (**ACTH**): A hormone released from a gland in the brain (**the pituitary**) and which controls the nutrition and growth of the part of the **adrenal gland** known as the adrenal cortex.

AIDS—acquired immune deficiency syndrome: Follows infection by a particular type of retrovirus called **HIV**. There may be a long period between exposure and development of clinical features. The clinical features include marked wasting of the muscles, recurrent infections, unusual skin cancers, and, in most cases, death.

Amino acids: These are the building blocks from which proteins are constructed (in technical terms they are organic acids in which one of the hydrogen atoms has been replaced).

Animal models: Animals which either spontaneously, or, following exposure to foreign material, develop the signs, symptoms, and blood test abnormalities which resemble a human disease.

Ankylosing spondylitis: A disease more common in men. Starting as stiffness in the lower back, it may involve the whole of the spine.

Antibody: A form of protein in the blood **serum** or **plasma**. Antibodies are usually formed in response to the presence of an **antigen**.

Antigen: Any of various types of material (including micro-organisms, foreign proteins, and others) that as a result of coming into contact with appropriate tissues or an animal body can stimulate an immune response after a short period.

Antinuclear antibody: A type of antibody that binds to a protein in the nucleus of the cell—usually **DNA, RNA,** or some other protein component of the nucleus. (Although low levels of such antibodies may be present in some healthy normal people, especially the elderly, these antibodies are usually found in patients with autoimmune diseases.)

Apheresis: Process of removing blood or some component of it from the body.

Arachidonic acid: A breakdown product of phospholipids which may be converted into a variety of **prostaglandins** or **leucotrienes**.

Arthritis: Inflammation of a joint usually associated with pain and swelling. Over 200 forms of arthritis exist.

Asthma: A disease characterized by recurrent attacks of shortness of breath due to a reversible spasm (reduction in size) of the small bronchial tubes.

Autoantibodies: Antibodies which bind to components of the body's own tissues.

Autoimmune: A disordered response of the immune system directed against a constituent of the individual's own body.

Azathioprine: A drug which suppresses the immune system. It has been used since the 1960s, when it was introduced to help prevent the rejection of transplanted organs into the body.

B cell (B lymphocyte): A type of **lymphocyte** which has not been processed in the thymus gland but in other parts of the lymphatic tissues (in birds these cells are processed in an organ known as the Bursa of Fabricius—hence the name).

Bacteria: Any type of small micro-organism consisting of just one cell.

Basophils: A form of white cell (**leucocyte**) characterized by the relatively pale, amoeba-like nucleus and large, coarse granules.

Cancer: A general term used to indicate the uncontrolled overgrowth of cells. Most cancers are characterized by a tendency to invade adjacent tissues or to spread to distant sites. Many cancers are potentially fatal.

Carbohydrate: Molecules usually made up of varying amounts of carbon, hydrogen, and oxygen forming a wide variety of sugar molecules such as starch and cellulose.

Cartilage: Part of the connective tissues of the body which has a firm consistency but few blood vessels. It consists of a mixture of cells and the material, or matrix, in which they are embedded.

Cell membrane: The outer cell membrane separates the inner contents of the cell from its surroundings. The membrane is usually composed of fats or lipids and regulates the passage of fluids and other materials in and out of the cell. Inner cell membranes surround and separate individual components of the cell.

Cerebrospinal fluid: The fluid which bathes the brain and spinal cord.

Chromosome: A constituent of the cell nucleus that carries the genes. It changes shape during the lifetime of the cell and is capable of reproducing the cell's physical and clinical structure through successive cell divisions.

Clonal deletion: The removal of particular **clones** of cells, usually **lymphocytes,** which usually takes place in the thymus gland. It is an important mechanism to remove potentially harmful cells.

Clonal expansion: The encouragement of particular **clones** of cells, usually **lymphocytes,** to increase in numbers usually for the purpose of helping to defend the body against invading organisms.

Clone: A group of identical cells all of which come from an original single cell.

Coeliac disease: A condition usually beginning in childhood or early adult life in which the gut is unable to absorb food, especially fat, properly into the bloodstream. The results include passing motions with a very strong smell that have a high fat content, muscle weakness, and generalized wasting of the body.

Complement: A heat-sensitive group of proteins in normal serum that are important for the removal of bacteria and other cells thought to be harmful to the body.

Concordance rate: A term usually used in the study of the genetics of twins to indicate the frequency with which a particular disease has occurred in both.

Control populations: A term usually employed as a comparison when studying the occurrence of diseases in particular groups of individuals. (The control populations need to be matched for age and sex with the study group.)

Corticosteroids: Chemical substances which can occur naturally as hormones produced from the adrenal cortex situated just above the kidneys. They may also be manufactured and used to block, in part, the damaging effects of autoimmunity.

Crohn's disease: A particular type of inflammation of the gut. It may affect any part of the gut, from mouth to anus; the inflammation has been principally found beneath the lining surface of the gut. The cause of this condition is unknown.

Cyclosporin (A): Derived originally from a fungus this drug has powerful effects suppressing the immune system and is now widely used to prevent the rejection of transplanted organs.

Cytokines: These are small proteins produced by various cells which have many important functions including control over cells of the immune system, blocking the effects of viruses and stimulating the growth of blood and other cells.

Demyelination: A process in which the outer lining sheath of nerve cells is stripped away preventing the efficient passage of electrical discharges. This process is largely responsible for the damage done to the nervous system in patients with multiple sclerosis.

Dendritic cells: These cells are found throughout the body and have an amoeba-like appearance. These are mainly concerned with presenting captured antigen to the immune system.

Diabetes: A disease occurring in two forms (either diabetes mellitus or diabetes insipidus) which have in common a tendency to produce urine with a high sugar content. These conditions are associated with abnormalities of cells in the pancreas.

DNA (deoxyribonucleic acid): A large complex molecule which makes up the genetic code and the reproductive component of chromosomes and some **viruses**. It may exist in individual strands (single stranded) or paired strands (double-stranded), the strands being linked like the steps of a ladder.

Enzymes: Proteins secreted by the body cells that help to induce chemical changes in other substances whilst remaining apparently unchanged in the process.

Eosinophil: A form of white cell which stains with eosin dyes.

Epstein–Barr virus: A virus that, in the West, is known to be responsible for glandular fever (infectious mononucleosis). In China it is thought to be responsible for the much more serious nasal pharyngeal cancer. Some believe it may be the trigger to the development of rheumatoid arthritis and in Africa for a form of lymphoma, a cancer of the **lymph** glands.

Erythrocytes: Red blood cells.

Fatty acid: Any form of acid which combines with glycerine to form fat. These acids are subdivided into saturated, meaning that the carbon atoms within the acid are connected by single bonds, or unsaturated, in which the carbon chains contain one or more double or triple bonds.

Gammaglobulin: A protein fraction of the serum that comprises the majority of **immunoglobulins** and **antibodies**.

Genes: Small segments of a **chromosome** which code for specific proteins and are capable of reproducing themselves exactly at each cell division.

Genetic engineering: The manipulation of **genes** to cause a change in the protein product they provide a blue-print for. There is much interest at present in manipulating (i.e. replacing or removing) potentially harmful genes such as those which cause the disease cystic fibrosis.

Glycosylation: A process by which **carbohydrate** molecules are added to proteins.

Goodpasture's syndrome: A rare condition associated with inflammation in the kidneys and lungs.

Granulocyte: A mature white blood cell, which may be a **neutrophil**, an **eosinophil**, or a **basophil**.

Graves' disease: A condition due to over activity of the thyroid gland associated with overproduction of the **hormone,** thyroxine. It often results in a fast heart rate, weight loss, and bulging, staring eyes.

Haemoglobin: An essential **protein** present in red blood cells that is capable of transporting oxygen from the lungs to the tissues.

Haemolytic anaemia: An **autoimmune** disease in which the body's immune system destroys its own red cells.

Hashimoto's disease: An **autoimmune** disease in which the thyroid gland becomes relatively inactive causing dryness of the skin and hair, swelling of the gland itself, and a general feeling of fatigue.

Heat shock proteins: Different families of proteins which have survived, often in very similar forms, through evolution and which have two main functions. First, they have important roles in the normal cell acting for example as chaperones of other proteins being moved around the cell. Second, they have important protective value to the cell when it is exposed to excess heat and other forms of stress.

Hiatus hernia: A condition in which the upper part of the stomach has a tendency to pass through the diaphragm muscle into the upper chest. The consequence is that the acid contents of the stomach spill into the lower end of the oesophagus (the tube connecting the mouth to the stomach) causing a burning pain in the centre of the chest.

Histamine: A chemical present in ergot and in animal tissues which is both a powerful stimulant of cells in the lining of the stomach and, when pricked into the skin, causes a local increase in size of the blood vessels and fall in blood pressure.

HIV (human immunodeficiency virus): The agent responsible for causing **AIDS** and related disorders.

HLA (human leucocyte antigens): These are molecules, coded by different genes and present on the surface of many cells, that are essential in mounting a normal immune response.

Hormones: Chemical substances formed in one organ or part of the body and carried in the blood to another organ enabling it to function normally.

Idiotype: Part of an **antibody** which may itself stimulate the production of another antibody to itself (known as the anti-idiotype).

Immune complex: A combination of an **antigen** and an **antibody.** Such complexes are formed as part of the normal functioning of the **immune system,** but may on occasion contribute to the development of an **autoimmune** disease.

Immune response: The way in which the **immune system** acts when challenged by the presence of a foreign unaltered self-antigen. In the first instance **immunoglobulin** M (IgM) **antibodies** are produced to the **antigen** but later immunoglobulin G (IgG) antibodies are made.

Immune system: The sophisticated network of cells, principally **lymphocytes,** and their products such as **antibodies** and organs (mainly the liver, bone marrow, and spleen) that provide a form of constant radar for the body to identify foreign 'invaders' and the means to destroy them.

Immunity: A state in which the body acquires protection against an infectious agent or one of its products. This may occur naturally; for example the immunity that follows infection with measles or artificially as occurs after vaccination against diphtheria.

Immunodeficiency: A general term implying that the immune system is in some way defective. This may be due to an inherited defect, as occurs with certain complement deficiencies, or as an acquired defect as may occur following exposure to HIV.

Immunoglobulins: Proteins linked to **carbohydrate** that function as **antibodies.**

Immunosuppressive drugs: Drugs that are capable of suppressing the **immune response.** Most were initially introduced for the treatment of various forms of cancer and to prevent transplanted organs from being rejected but have also been found to be helpful in the treatment of many types of **autoimmune** disease.

Inflammation: The response of the body to injury or abnormal stimulation (caused by a physical, chemical, or biological agent). The consequence is swelling, redness, pain, and local heat.

Inoculation: The process of preventing a 'full blown' disease by injections of micro-organisms or material derived from them which have been rendered safe.

Interferons: A group of small **proteins** produced by infected host cells that protect non-infected cells from viral infection.

Interleukins: Cytokines that are produced by **leucocytes** and are active in inflammation.

Klinefelter syndrome: A rare condition seen in men who have an additional X chromosome and who have underdeveloped male sexual characteristics with some breast swelling and a low sperm count.

Langerhans' cells: Specialized cells found in the skin, lungs, and pancreas gland.

Leucocyte: Any one of the white blood cells. They may be found in the bone marrow, liver, or spleen and are subdivided into several types.

Leucotrienes: Breakdown products of a form of saturated fatty acid that have the ability to dilate blood vessels.

Leukaemia: Malignant condition (**cancer**) of the cells that produce white blood cells.

Lipids: A term used to describe fats and oils.

Lumbar puncture: A procedure in which a needle is inserted at the base of the spine into the space containing the cerebrospinal fluid. The procedure is most often used to analyse the contents of cerebrospinal fluid, but may sometimes be used as a means of delivering drugs direct to the central nervous system.

Lymph: Fluid that is collected from tissues throughout the body flowing in the lymphatic vessels through the lymph nodes eventually added to the venous blood circulation.

Lymphocytes: A type of white blood cell formed in lymphoid tissues throughout the body such as lymph nodes, spleen, and thymus.

Macroglobulinaemia: The presence in the blood of a particular type of **protein**, known as **gammaglobulin**, which is unusually large. These are often found in patients with a **multiple myeloma**, in which there is widespread destruction of the bone marrow.

Macrophages: Large white blood cells with a single nucleus found in many tissues and organs of the body; often concerned with the removal of dead cells or foreign material.

Magnetic resonance imaging (**MRI**): An imaging procedure that depends upon the behaviour of certain nuclei in a magnetic field. In the presence of large magnets the nuclei may resonate, and the intensity of the signal produced can be converted to a visual image. The principle was initially discovered in 1946 and used first as an analytical tool in physics and chemistry. In the past ten years a new form of imaging has been invented, which provides visual images of quite stunning clarity. MRI scanners are now widely available in hospitals throughout the world.

Major histocompatibility complex (MHC): Genes located on the short arm of the **chromosome** that determines which **antigens** are found on the surfaces of the cells of the body.

Malignant: The term applied to a cancerous growth or neoplasm often resistant to treatment.

Mast cells: Cells, found in the tissues, which contain rather coarse **basophilic** granules that can be stained using basic dyes.

6-Mercaptopurine: An immunosuppressive drug used in the treatment of some forms of **cancer**. Its use in the treatment of **autoimmune** disease has been replaced by its 'close relation', **azathioprine**.

Metabolism: The sum of chemical changes whereby food that is eaten is used to convert either small molecules into larger ones, e.g. **amino acids** into **protein** (anabolism), or large molecules into smaller ones, e.g. protein into amino acids (catabolism).

Molecular mimicry: A term referring to an identical or very similar group of **amino acids** found in otherwise very different **proteins**. A possible consequence is that an **antibody** directed against the sequence of amino acids would bind to two apparently distinct proteins.

Monoclonal antibodies: Identical antibodies produced from a single **clone** of cells. Although they can occur naturally, monoclonal antibodies are usually the result of a fusion between a form of **cancer** cell and an **antibody**-producing **lymphocyte**. The cancer cell provides **genes** which encode for potential immortality and the **lymphocyte** cell provides the genes and produces antibodies. Using suitable purification techniques, large amounts of **immunoglobulin** with a single type of reactivity can be produced. Since the discovery of this process some twenty years ago, monoclonal antibodies have been used widely to identify particular **antigens** and, more recently, as therapeutic agents.

Multiple myeloma: A form of **cancer** of the **B cells** (i.e. the **lymphocytes** that produce **antibodies**).

Multiple sclerosis: Disease of the nervous system, generally occurring early in adult life, which results in damage to the myelinated nerves. It may cause a variety of clinical features including paralysis, tremor, and disturbances of speech and/or vision.

Myasthenia gravis: An uncommon **autoimmune** muscle disease due to loss of **acetylcholine receptors**. Myasthenia gravis causes an inability to sustain a muscle contraction (thus the eyelids of a patient asked to gaze up at the ceiling will begin to droop after a short time).

Myelin: The sheath which surrounds many nerve cells and enables the rapid passage of a nerve impulse.

Myeloma: Tumour of the antibody-producing cells.

Myositis: An inflammatory condition of skeletal muscle more common in women between the ages of 30 to 50, which may on occasion be accompanied by a skin rash (dermatomyositis) over the eyelids and outer surfaces of the arms.

Neutrophils: Mature white blood cells formed in the bone marrow, present in the circulating blood, they are involved in the process of **inflammation** (see also **granulocytes**).

Oncogenes: Genes responsible for a predisposition towards the development of malignancy.

Osteoarthritis: A condition of the synovial joints characterized by the loss of **cartilage** often accompanied by new bone formation in areas adjacent to the cartilage loss.

Osteoporosis: The reduction in bone mass and strength often occurring in women after the menopause. It results in increased risk of fracture with little or even no trauma.

Pancreas: Gland found in the abdomen, surrounded by the bowel, which secretes a substance required in the digestion of food. It also secretes the **hormone** insulin, which controls the level of glucose in the blood.

Pannus: The type of tissue found at the junction between the cartilage, bone, and synovium in patients with **rheumatoid arthritis**. This tissue can invade the **cartilage** and bone, causing erosion.

Parasite: An organism that lives on or in another organism and which draws its nourishment from (and thereby causes damage to) its host.

Parathyroid: Small glands situated close to the thyroid gland in the neck which are responsible for regulating the level of calcium in the body.

Pathogenesis: Process by which diseases develop.

Pathology: The branch of medical science dealing with all aspects of disease, especially their causes and the processes which lead to them.

Pemphigus: An **autoimmune** disease characterized by skin blisters.

Phagocytosis: The process by which white cells surround and digest pieces of dead and dying tissue, bacteria, foreign particles, etc.

Pituitary gland: A small but most important gland situated in the brain, which secretes a wide variety of hormones controlling growth and the normal functioning of the thyroid and adrenal glands amongst others.

Plasma: The fluid part of the blood (see also **serum**).

Plasma cells: Fully formed **antibody**-synthesizing cells that are derived from **B cells**.

Plasma exchange (plasmapheresis): The mechanism by which blood is taken from an individual and split into the cellular and **plasma** components. The patient's plasma is replaced with plasma from a healthy individual and the resulting blood mixture (the patient's own cellular components and the new plasma) is returned to the patient. This technique was widely used in the 1970s and 1980s; however, its effectiveness in most **autoimmune** diseases is doubted now.

Platelets: Cells present in the blood lacking a nucleus but enabling the blood to clot.

Polyclonal activation: A stimulus for several or many types of **B cell** (at much the same time) causing the increased production of different sorts of **antibodies**.

Polyreactivity: The ability of an **antibody** to bind to seemingly different **proteins** or glycoproteins. This may be because the apparently different structures actually have an identical small section or because the antibody can recognize different structures on different **antigens**.

Predisposition: Increased tendency to develop a particular disease.

Prevalence: Term used to describe the numbers of current cases of a particular disease at a particular point in time. It may be used in a cumulative sense over a fixed period.

Primary biliary cirrhosis: An **autoimmune** disease affecting the liver —

more common in women—which may result in jaundice and attacks of abdominal pain.

Prostaglandins: A variety of small, naturally occurring acidic compounds with a variety of biological activities, which include increasing the permeability of blood vessels, increasing the contraction of certain muscle cells, and reducing the size of the small bronchial tubes. Prostaglandins also cause immune stimulation and suppression.

Proteins: A complex group of substances, principally made up of **amino acids**, and constituting the greater parts of the nitrogen-containing components of animal and vegetable tissue.

Raynaud's phenomenon: Named after the French physician who described a characteristic colour change—white to blue to red—in the fingers and toes, and sometimes on the tip of the nose and ears, in response to a change in temperature usually from hot to cold. In some patients emotional distress can have the same effect.

Red blood cells (**erythrocytes**): Formed in the bone marrow, their major function is to carry oxygen from the lungs to the tissues.

Relative risk: Term used to compare the chances of an individual with a given set of genes developing a particular disease compared with another individual who lacks these same genes.

Retrovirus: RNA viruses that reproduce themselves via an intermediate under the control of a particular **enzyme** known as reverse transcriptase.

Rheumatoid arthritis: A disease that usually starts in the small joints of the hands and feet. Common in women, it most often begins between the ages of 30 and 55. There are several types; some patients make a full recovery but others suffer major joint destruction.

Rheumatoid factor: A type of **antibody** which binds to a particular site of **immunoglobulin** G. Rheumatoid factor may be found in healthy people but it is present in high level in patients with **rheumatoid arthritis**. Also known as a self-associating antibody.

Rifampicin: A drug used in the treatment of tuberculosis.

RNA (**ribonucleic acid**): **DNA** acts as a template for the production of RNA, which in turn acts as a template for the production of **proteins** in the cell.

Scleroderma: Literally 'hard skin'. This is a most unpleasant disease, mainly confined to women, in which greatly increased amounts of collagen form in the skin causing it to thicken and harden. The same process may also involve the internal organs, mostly the heart, lungs, and kidneys.

Serum: The fluid part of the blood (that which is obtained after the blood coagulates).

Sjögren's syndrome: Named after Henrik Sjögren, Swedish ophthalmologist. It is characterized by dryness of the eyes and mouth in association with inflammation of the glands which usually secrete fluid to keep these organs moist.

SLE (systemic lupus erythematosus): A disease largely confined to women during child-bearing years, which is characterized by a very wide variety of clinical features especially skin rashes, fatigue, swelling of the **lymph** glands, and inflammation of the heart, lungs, kidneys, and central nervous system. It is also associated with many blood test abnormalities especially the presence of **antibodies** to **DNA**.

Spondylitis: Inflammation of one or more of the tissues that link the vertebrae.

Stem cells: Primitive cells which develop into the different types of white blood cells, red blood cells, etc.

Surface markers: The structures found on the outside of cells which usually differ between cell types and are usually under genetic control.

Susceptibility: Term used in the general medical sense to refer to the risk of developing a given disease.

Synovial joints: Joints lined by a particular type of membrane which secretes a fluid lubricating the joint and the surfaces of a related tendon.

T cell (T lymphocyte): A **thymus**-derived cell that takes part in a wide variety of **immune** reactions.

T cytotoxic (killer) cell: A type of **T cell** that is directly damaging to other cells or tissues.

T helper cell: A variety of **T cell** that 'helps' or stimulates **B cells** to produce **antibody**.

T suppressor cell: A form of **T cell** that acts to stop **B cells** from producing **antibodies**.

Tetracycline: A widely available form of antibiotic.

Thrombocytopenia: A reduction in the number of circulating platelet cells.

Thymoma: A form of tumour of the thymus gland often associated with **myasthenia gravis**.

Thymus: A lymphoid organ (see **lymph**) found in the lower part of the neck. It plays an essential role in the development of the immune system by acting as the site for the processing of newly formed **lymphocytes** and the removal of most of those that could be harmful to the body.

Thyroiditis: Literally inflammation of the thyroid gland, which is often due to an **autoimmune** process. This may result in the reduced production of the thyroid hormone, causing a generalized slowing down of the body's metabolism or, on occasions, may stimulate the production of this hormone, leading to an increased body metabolism.

Thyrotoxicosis: Over-activity of the thyroid gland usually due to the excessive stimulation or receptor for the thyroid hormone. The condition causes an increased pulse rate, a wide-eyed appearance, and a feeling of anxiety, among other symptoms (see also **Graves' disease**).

Tissue typing: An assessment of the human leucocyte antigens (**HLA**) present in different individuals in order to determine their suitability for organ transplant as either donor or receiver.

Trimolecular complex: The combination of **antigen** in the form of a peptide presented together with **HLA** class 1 molecules to a **T cell** receptor. By this mechanism a wide variety of antigens is processed by the body's **immune system**.

Tumour necrosis factors (TNF): A class of **cytokines** usually devided into TNFalpha and TNFbeta. TNF alpha is known to play a major role in inducing **inflammation**.

Ulcerative colitis: **Inflammation** of the lining of the lower part of the bowel causing loss of blood through the anus and often abdominal pain.

Uveitis: **Inflammation** of the part of the eye known as the uveal tract, consisting of the iris and adjacent structures. This inflammation may also be part of an **autoimmune** response.

Vaccine: Classically a modified form of micro-organism incapable of producing a severe infection but able to stimulate the **immune system** to provide protection against the 'real' organism. The use of the term has now been broadened to include various synthetic products.

Virus: A term for a group of potentially pathogenic organisms which are invisible under the ordinary microscope and which consist of minute particles of **RNA** or **DNA**. They have the ability to cause disease in plants, bacteria, insects, animal, and man: they are capable of passing through fine filters that retain bacteria.

X-ray: A form of electromagnetic radiation that can pass through solid bodies and is used as both an imaging technique and, at much higher doses, as a form of treatment for various forms of **cancer**.

Index